# Nurse Edith Cavell

# Nurse Edith Cavell

Two Accounts of a Notable British Nurse
of the First World War

The Martyrdom of Nurse Cavell
William Thomson Hill

With Edith Cavell in Belgium
Jacqueline Van Til

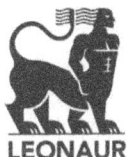

LEONAUR

*Nurse Edith Cavell*
*Two Accounts of a Notable British Nurse*
*of the First World War*
*The Martyrdom of Nurse Cavell* by William Thomson Hill
and
*With Edith Cavell in Belgium* by Jacqueline Van Til

First published under the titles
*The Martyrdom of Nurse Cavell*
and
*With Edith Cavell in Belgium*

Leonaur is an imprint of Oakpast Ltd

Copyright in this form © 2011 Oakpast Ltd

ISBN: 978-0-85706-507-0 (hardcover)
ISBN: 978-0-85706-508-7 (softcover)

http://www.leonaur.com

# Contents

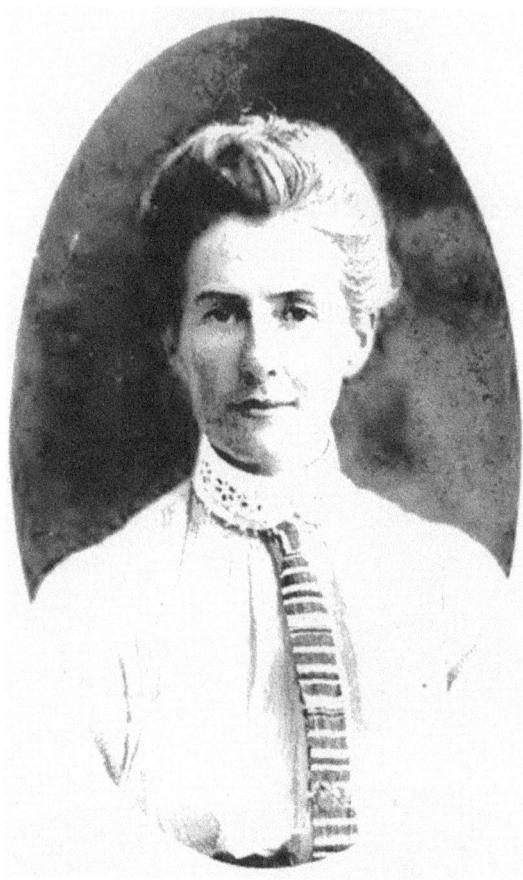

Nurse Edith Cavell

# The Martyrdom of Nurse Cavell

William Thomson Hill

# Contents

NURSE CAVELL'S LAST MESSAGE TO THE WORLD.

*But this I would say,*
*standing as I do in view of God and eternity,*
*I realise that patriotism is not enough.*
*I must have no hatred or bitterness to anyone.*

# CHAPTER 1

# Childhood

In the early seventies there were living at the country rectory of Swardeston, near Norwich, a clergyman and his wife and little family. There was a "New" and an "Old" Rectory. Both are still standing, much as they were then, except that the trees are older, and the "New" Rectory has long ago lost any signs of newness. It is one of the ways of Old England to call some of its most ancient things New, as if it could never learn to tolerate change kindly, even after centuries of wont.

There is a Newtimber Place in Sussex whose walls were built before the Armada. There is a New Building in Peterborough Cathedral which was completed before the Reformation. New Shoreham took the place of Old Shoreham before Magna Charta was signed.

The Rector, the Rev. Frederick Cavell, lived with his family at the New Rectory. It is a pleasant sunny house with a large garden. Such parsonages are common in all the unspoiled rural parts of England. A little gate leads to the churchyard close by.

In a great city no man would live willingly close by a cemetery. In such a village as Swardeston the nearness of the graveyard is a consecration. New graves appear among the old ones from time to time. The oldest of these others have faded gently into the grass. Nobody is left to tend them or to remember whose bones they cover. Yet the history of many a family can be traced back for three centuries on the lichen-covered stones.

Some day, when the war is over, another grave may be dug in this quiet spot. If the poor mutilated frame of Edith Cavell is ever permitted to be brought back home, her countrymen will come here to look upon the place where she lies. In this October of 1915 she sleeps in a land ravaged by war, and those who killed her will not stoop even to the tardy pity of giving back her body.

But in those early seventies the village churchyard was not a place of sadness to the Rectory children. They played hide-and-seek among the sloping tombstones. The church and churchyard were, as they still are, the centre of the village life. Gay doings, such as a wedding, took place under the shadows of the elms and yews.

The whole community assembled there on any day of special interest. The churchyard was the Trafalgar Square of Swardeston. For it was not remote from the houses, as many village churchyards are. Norfolk labourers swung their heels on the wall in the long evenings of the days before village institutes and reading rooms were invented.

In these early seventies the village talk still harked back sometimes to the War of the French and Prussians. Its politics dealt with such names as "Dizzy" and Gladstone and Joseph Arch, the agricultural reformer—and, what was more to the point, a Norfolk man. In later years the village church saw the celebrations of Queen Victoria's two Jubilees and King Edward's Coronation—"a Norfolk landlord, and a rare good 'un," as they liked to say in Swardeston.

CHAPTER 2

# Life in the Rectory

Home life in the Rectory was tinged, as was that of most English homes at the time, with Evangelical strictness. On Sunday all books, needlework, and toys were put away. The day began with the learning of collect or Catechism. As soon as the children were big enough they attended services in the morning and afternoon.

Evening services were not yet introduced in Swardeston. Light was not cheap, and the way across the country fields to church was no adventure for Sabbath clothes on dark winter nights. Thus the closing hours on Sunday were home hours for Rectory and village. Let those who have no memories of such times scoff if Edith Cavell's father was Rector of this parish for more than fifty years. He is dead now, but the villagers remember him well. His portrait shows him with a mouth and chin of unusual firmness. His eyes are kindly, but there is little sense of humour about them. It is notably the face of an upright man. Surely capable of sternness, he would be just to the point of inexorableness unless his face belies him. A sense of duty is implicit in every line; and we have the best of reasons for knowing that he transmitted this part of his character to his daughter Edith.

"The clever Miss Cavell" she was called in later years when she worked at a London hospital; but a more dominant characteristic was a rigid insistence upon what she deemed to be right. This was the constant theme of the father's sermons to his village flock. He would not hesitate to reproach from the pulpit any member of the congregation, whatever his station, whom he considered guilty of grave fault.

The mother, (who is now eighty years old, and lives very quietly at Norwich, [at time of first publication]), brought a gentler influence to bear upon the Rectory life. There is a picture of her with two of her little girls. The mother wears the wide flounces which today are among the earliest memories of the "Men of Forty." Flounces that were a protection and a promise. Something for little hands to cling to when the legs were not yet sure of their way. These flounces made a royal road from earth to the children's heaven. The grownup world far out of reach was always within call of a pull at the ample skirts.

Mrs. Cavell was a happy mother, and her children were happy too. So early as the days we are speaking of her eyes had something wistful in them. It was almost as if some inner consciousness had told her then of the distant, poignant future.

So the family grew up in a contented, well-ordered home, with plenty of outdoor games and sunshine, such as country children have. Long afterwards, in the midst of London slums, Edith Cavell would talk of the ripening blackberries far away in the Norfolk lanes, and of the great jam-making times which followed.

# CHAPTER 3

# Work in London

Like Charlotte Bronte, another vicar's daughter, Edith Cavell first learned something of the wider world in a Brussels school. It was commoner then than now—meaning by "now" before the war—for English girls to be sent to Belgium to school. Charlotte Bronte's Brussels life has left us at least one imperishable book. Edith Cavell has left no written memorials of those times; but if we would reconstruct her life we may imagine some such background as that of "Villette": the strangeness of a foreign city, fascinating by its novelty yet repelling by alien atmosphere.

The lot of a schoolgirl is not too happy at the best among new companions. When their language and ways are those of a foreign country they can become a source of torture to a sensitive child. Some of these schoolgirl irritations Edith Cavell had to bear; yet such early annoyances evidently left little mark on her, for she returned many years later to Brussels of her own free will, and conquered the affections of the Belgians a second time.

Edith Cavell's early womanhood was spent in London—at the London Hospital, the St. Pancras Infirmary, and the Shoreditch Infirmary in Hoxton. Her training was obtained at the London Hospital, the great institution in the Whitechapel Road which is now nursing many wounded soldiers, (at time of first publication). The women who train in this hospital pass through a hard school. All hospital nurses work hard, but the nurses who come from "The London" think they know more of the strain of their calling than any others.

"The London" proposes to raise a memorial to Nurse Cavell. It is their right and hers that this should be done. For "The London" gave her the thorough training which enabled her to become the skilful teacher of others, and to instruct the nurses who should succour with equal care the wounded of all nations.

At the end of her arduous training at the London Hospital in 1896, Miss Cavell went to St. Pancras Infirmary as Night Superintendent. She stayed there for a little more than three years. Then she became Assistant Matron at the Shoreditch Infirmary in Hoxton. She left Hoxton in 1906 to start the work in Brussels which ended only with her cruel death.

Including the training years at the London Hospital, Edith Cavell had given twenty-two years to nursing the sick. She was twenty-one years old when she began this work. She was forty-three when she met her death. Thus she had given up the best years of a woman's life without a break, save for the occasional precious holidays, of which we shall say a word presently.

The work in London was one of unvarying routine in the most dismal surroundings. Nothing but a real devotion to the task could have made the monotony tolerable.

The writer asked one of those who worked with her for part of this time what was the reason that decided Edith Cavell to become a nurse. "She felt it was her vocation," was the simple answer; "isn't that enough?" The vocation, in these great London infirmaries, consisted in preserving a cheerful face day in and day out; in ruling, with kindness but also with firmness and an unfaltering tact, old men and women, children from the poorest slums; in being constantly in contact with pain and suffering and in the near presence of death. Those who remember her work in London—and they are very many—speak of her unselfishness and of a shy pride about the details of her labours.

What she did for her patients she liked to be a secret between herself and them.

She would follow up the "cases" to their homes. The matron and her fellow-nurses guessed some of these acts of weekday holiness; but Nurse Cavell never spoke of them. She went about doing good among the neat beds of the wards and in the unlovely surroundings of the neighbouring streets, doubtless thinking sometimes of the Norfolk village where the sun was shining beyond the fog, yet never letting the patients see that she had any thoughts except for them.

But with this sympathy went a rare strength of mind. Her name "Clever Miss Cavell" was not used in envy. It was a simple recognition of the fact that she had what is called a capable brain. She always knew what to do in a difficult situation. A fellow-nurse in trouble was always advised to consult Miss Cavell.

# CHAPTER 4

# Uphill Work in Brussels

Edith Cavell needed all her strength of character in her first years in Brussels. When she went there nine years ago as matron of a Surgical and Medical Home, English nursing methods were not appreciated on the Continent as they are now. Nursing was regarded as one of the functions of the Church. Miss Cavell was a Protestant as well as a foreigner. She was felt to be a rival of the nuns and sisters working under religious vows.

The authorities of the Catholic Church looked coldly upon an enterprise which, from their point of view, had an aspect of irreligion and freethinking. But it was not long before the matron's efficiency and tact carried the day. A well-known priest trusted himself to the English lady. His tribute to her devotion and skill brought public opinion to her side. In 1909 she established a training home for nurses. The authorities recognised and encouraged her; and shortly before the outbreak of war she was provided with a modern and well-equipped building.

The first warning of the war came when she was spending a holiday at home with her mother at Norwich. During these years in Brussels two holidays a year had been spent in England. They were happy halting places in a rough journey. What made them so pleasant to Edith Cavell was that she could spend them with her mother.

The love of the younger woman for the old was one of the most beautiful aspects of her character. "People may look upon me as a lonely old maid," she said once to a friend; "but with a mother like mine to look after, and, in addition, my work in the world which I love, I am such a happy old maid that everyone would feel envious of me if they only knew."

That was her secret—her love for her mother and her work. It was

19

that which enabled her to look upon the world as a beautiful garden, where there was always something to do for sickly plants. The real flowers, and the care of them which could only be given in English holidays, were almost a passion to her from the earliest Rectory days.

Her success as a nurse, both in Brussels and the slums of London, owed three-parts of its efficacy to her overflowing sympathy. "It was her gentle way," said an old patient, "that did most to make me well again; I felt she was a minister of God working for my good." And there are wounded British soldiers who have pressed the doctors to send them back quickly to the firing line. "We will go back willingly," they say, "to avenge this great woman's death."

Every holiday in England was spent with the aged mother, who looked forward to these meetings as much as the daughter. Without warning, the war broke into the last of these holidays in the full summer of 1914. Edith Cavell made her mind up promptly. Her holiday was not yet over, but she hurried back at once. "My duty is out there," she said; "I shall be wanted."

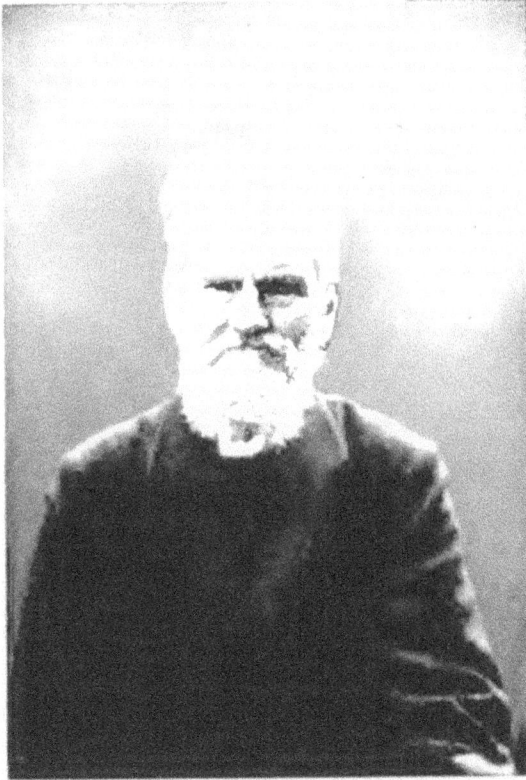

THE REV. FREDERICK CAVELL,
FATHER OF NURSE CAVELL

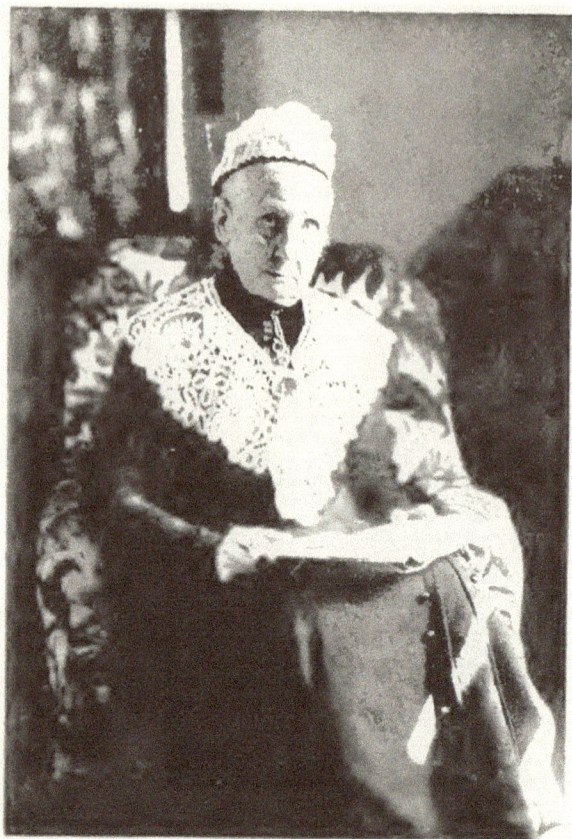

Mrs. Cavell, Mother of Nurse Cavell

## Chapter 5

# The Coming of the Germans

We reach now the last year of Edith Cavell's life, for which all the others had been a preparation. When she arrived in Brussels, the Germans were shelling Liége. The gallant little Belgium Army stood drawn up across the path of the invaders. It was believed that the French and British would soon arrive to drive the Germans back. The Belgian Government was still in Brussels. Cheery Burgomaster Max kept order with his Civic Guard. In the autumn of 1915 we are all wiser.

Miss Cavell has herself described, in an article sent home to the *Nursing Mirror*, how the bitter truth came home to Brussels:—

Brussels lay that evening (August 20th) breathless with anxiety. News came that the Belgians, worn-out and weary, were unable to hold back the oncoming host who might be with us that night. Still we clung to the hope that the English Army was between us and the unseen peril. . . .

In the evening came the news that the enemy were at the gates. At midnight bugles were blowing, summoning the Civic Guard to lay down their arms and leave the city. Many people were up through the dark hours, and all doors and windows were tightly shut. As we went to bed our only consolation was that in God's good time right and justice must prevail.

The sympathies of Nurse Cavell were all with the Belgians and their Allies. How could it be otherwise? Yet, when the Germans came she spoke with sympathy of the tired and footsore men in the enemy's host:—

On August 21st (she wrote) many more troops came through;

from our road we could see the long procession, and when the halt was called at midday and carts came up with supplies some were too weary to eat, and slept on the pavement of the street. We were divided between pity for these poor fellows far from their country and their people, suffering the weariness and fatigue of an arduous campaign, and hate of a cruel and vindictive foe bringing ruin and desolation on hundreds of happy homes and to a prosperous and peaceful land.

Some of the Belgians spoke to the invaders in German, and found they were very vague as to their whereabouts and imagined they were already in Paris; they were surprised to be speaking to Belgians, and could not understand what quarrel they had with them.

I saw several of the men pick up little children and give them chocolate or seat them on their horses, and some had tears in their eyes at the recollection of the little ones at home.

From that date till now we have been cut off from the world.

. . .

The German nurses training under Miss Cavell had already left— conducted to the frontier by her to save them the anxiety of being in an enemy capital. At this time the German soldiers were ruthlessly slaughtering Belgian women and children. The new authorities approved of her continuing her work: no longer, since the outbreak of war, a training institution, but a Red Cross Hospital. It is admitted even by her enemies that she threw herself ardently into her work without respect of nationality. Wounded Belgians and Germans were treated alike. Many German officers passed through her hands.

There is now in hospital in England, (at time of first publication), a wounded Belgian who knew Miss Cavell in Brussels in those first days of the German occupation, and who speaks of the universal affection in which she was held.

CHAPTER 6

# Weaving the Net

The full story of the next few months of Edith Cavell's life cannot be told until after the war is over. Brussels, as she had written, became cut off from the world. The hospitable old city became a nest of spies. Newspapers were first stopped, then suppressed, and are now printed under German auspices. The few trains that run for passengers are in German hands, and wherever you go you must have, and pay for, a passport. No one speaks to his neighbour in the tram, for he may be a spy. Besides, what news is there to tell, and who has the heart to gossip, and what fashions are there to speak of, and who ever goes to a concert or a theatre nowadays, and who would care to tell of their all-absorbing anxiety as to how to make ends meet and spin out the last of the savings, or to keep the little mouths at home filled, with the stranger close by?"

The frank, open nature of Edith Cavell was ill-fitted for such an atmosphere of fear and deception. Everyone was "suspect," as in the days of the Paris Terror in 1793. It was enough, as then, to fall under "suspicion of being suspect." Edith Cavell was suspected, and cunning men sought how they might weave a net of accusation around her.

Nurse Cavell was an Englishwoman. That, was the beginning of her offence. I am not here to say she did no wrong. The full significance of her own brave admissions cannot yet be revealed. Her crime was the crime of humanity. The beginning of her offence, to the suspicious German mind, was that she was English and was popular. Everyone spoke of her untiring kindness and unfailing courage. It was enough. She must be dangerous, or all the world would not speak well of her. Nobody spoke well of the German governors of Brussels.

There is reason to believe that Miss Cavell came in contact, once at least, with the terrible Baron Von Bissing, the Governor-General. He

25

formed a strong opinion of her capacity and dauntless courage. The same head that contrived her secret trial and execution, directed, there is little reason to doubt, the weaving of the web that ensnared her. The cleverest spies in Von Bissing's service were set to watch her. They found out that she had given a greatcoat to a French soldier who afterwards escaped across the Dutch frontier. On another occasion she had given an exhausted Englishman a glass of water. Then the spies said, what was likely enough, that she had given money to Belgians, and that this had enabled them to escape.

In every part of the world these would be simple acts of humanity—for the suspicious Von Bissing they were crimes. "This must be stopped," he ordered.

# CHAPTER 7

# Arrest and Silence

Early in the evening of the 5th of August, a loud knock came to the door of Nurse Cavell's hospital in the *Rue de la Culture*. Five heavily-footed German soldiers and a corporal stood outside with a police officer. At that very moment the nurse was changing the bandages of a wounded German. The soldiers broke open the door with the butt-ends of their rifles, and rushed into the ward.

At a sign from the police officer—one of the creatures Von Bissing had set to watch the nurse's movements—the corporal seized Miss Cavell roughly. He tore out of her hand the lint with which she was about to bind the wounded man, and began to drag her away.

The Englishwoman, astonished but calm and dignified, asked for an explanation. The answer was a cuff. Von Bissing had not given instructions for any explanation. Nurse Cavell left her hospital for the last time, and was marched through the dark streets to the military prison of St. Gilles.

Three weeks of silence followed. Miss Cavell's friends in England knew nothing of her arrest. It was only by the good offices of a chance traveller from Belgium that the news reached the family near the end of August. At the request of the British Foreign Office, Dr. Page, American Ambassador in London, telegraphed for information to the American Minister in Brussels, Mr. Brand Whitlock.

The gaolers of Edith Cavell had used the interval well. It was decided, even before her arrest, that she was to be executed. But, first of all, seeing that the Louvain methods were grown obsolete, it was necessary to concoct a "case" against her. The spies had not done their work well enough. The greatcoat and the glass of water and the silver coins to hunted men were not sufficient for a conviction. There was only one method by which Edith Cavell could be convicted. That was from her own mouth.

In England when the meanest felon is arrested he is warned by the officer who reads the charge to him, that he need not make any statement unless he wishes, and that anything he says may be used in evidence against him. In Brussels, under German rule, Edith Cavell's judges deliberately set themselves to extort admissions by which to condemn her.

They refused her an advocate. They prevented communication with any soul who could give her counsel. They surrounded her arrest and imprisonment with secrecy lest any warning of her danger should reach her from outside. They contrived that she should be utterly alone.

To their astonishment they found their business easy. Miss Cavell gave them every help in her power. She had nothing to conceal, she said. She told them every incident which had a bearing on the charge. She supplied dates and details. Instead of the clumsy hearsay of the spies, her accusers had facts given them to build up a lengthy dossier. And when all was admitted it was nothing more than a series of acts of pity.

Those who think of this confession as a woman's weakness are in error. Edith Cavell was no ignorant girl. She well knew what she did. She would have been a better lawyer if she had refused to incriminate herself. She would have been a less noble woman. What she said she said to draw all the blame upon herself. Knowing well that death was the punishment, she did not shrink.

CHAPTER 8

# The False Friend

As Von Bissing had arrested Edith Cavell in secret, so he sought to judge her clandestinely. The trial took place before a court-martial on October 7th and 8th, with that of thirty-four other prisoners. Before this time Mr. Brand Whitlock, the American Minister, with his Secretary of Legation, Mr. Hugh Gibson, and his legal adviser, M. de Leval, a Belgian advocate, had stirred themselves actively on Miss Cavell's behalf. The story of how they were deliberately hoodwinked is one of the most ugly features of the case.

For ten days Baron Von der Lancken, the German Political Minister, sent no reply to Mr. Whitlock's appeal for information, and for authority to start the defence. Mr. Whitlock repeated his request on September 10th, but it was not until two days after this date that Baron Von der Lancken replied to the appeal. He set forth in this letter the only official statement ever made by the German authorities as to Miss Cavell's "crime." It is worth reading in his own words:—

> She has herself admitted that she concealed in her house French and English soldiers, as well as Belgians of military age, all desirous of proceeding to the front.
> She has also admitted having furnished these soldiers with the money necessary for their journey to France, and having facilitated their departure from Belgium by providing them with guides, who enabled them to cross the Dutch frontier secretly.
> Miss Cavell's defence is in the hands of the advocate Braun, who, I may add, is already in touch with the competent German authorities. In view of the fact that the Department of the Governor-General, as a matter of principle, does not allow accused persons to have any interviews whatever, I much regret

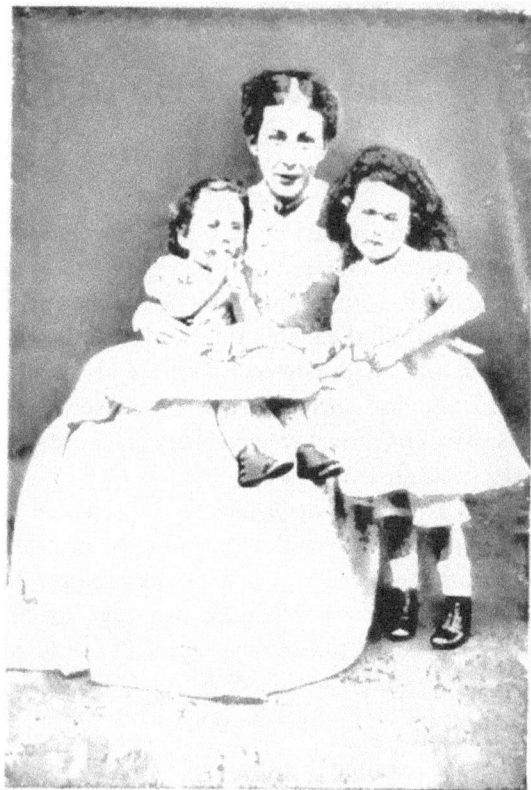

NURSE CAVELL WHEN A CHILD WITH HER
MOTHER AND ELDER SISTER

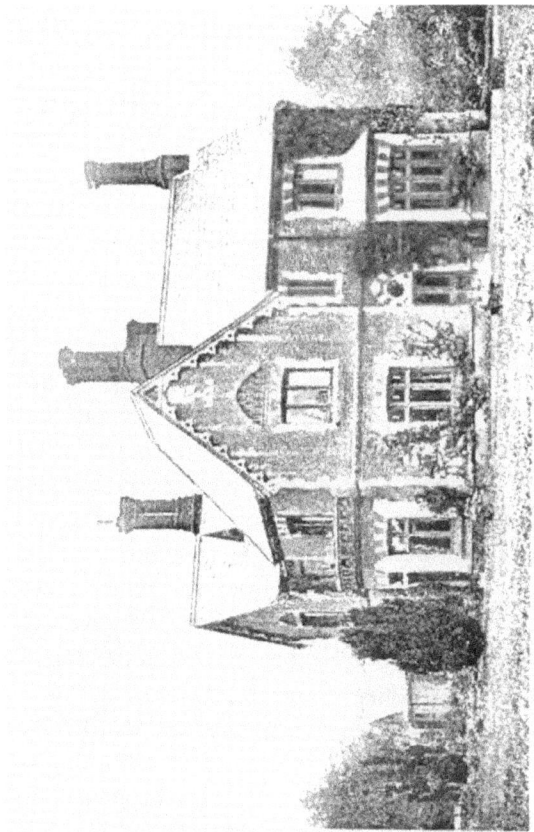

The Rectory at Swardeston, where Nurse Cavell was born

my inability to procure for Mr. de Leval permission to visit Miss Cavell as long as she is in solitary confinement.

Mr. Braun was a lawyer at the Brussels Appeal Court. As soon as the American Legation received the intimation that he had been appointed as the lawyer, Mr. de Leval wrote, asking him to come to the Legation. Mr. Braun came as requested "a few days later."

The time was now drawing close when the trial was to come on. Three weeks had already been wasted since the American Embassy in London first took the matter up, and nearly seven weeks had gone by since the arrest.

But when at last it appeared as though something was about to be done, another excuse was produced. Mr. Braun's news was that although he had been asked to defend Miss Cavell by personal friends of hers, he could not do so "owing to unforeseen circumstances."

Mr. Braun stated that he had seen another Belgian lawyer, Mr. Kirschen, who had agreed to undertake the defence. Another delay, while Mr. de Leval got into touch with Mr. Kirschen. At last there was to be an opportunity to obtain some details of the accusation. What had Miss Cavell admitted? asked the American counsel. What were the documents upon which the charge was based? What estimate had the lawyer formed of the prospects of an acquittal?

To the astonishment of Mr. de Leval, the lawyer replied that under German military rules he was not allowed to see his client before the trial began. The prosecution had every opportunity of preparing its case. The judges were fully informed of every circumstance that might bias them against the prisoner. But the poor lonely woman in prison could not even see her counsel in private, and all the documents were withheld from his inspection.

In these circumstances Mr. de Leval decided that he would attend the trial himself. Unfortunately, he did not persist in this decision.

It is extremely doubtful, in view of what happened afterwards, if the authorities would have permitted the presence of a neutral spectator of the administration of German "justice." What induced Mr. de Leval to give way was the consideration of Miss Cavell's interests. Mr. Kirschen urged that the presence of an American at the trial would prejudice the prisoner's chances. The judges would feel they were under supervision, and would be likely to be more severe in consequence. Mr. Kirschen declared that there was not the least chance of a miscarriage of justice, and promised to inform Mr. de Leval of every development of the case.

We may judge of the value of his advocacy from the fact that he afterwards broke all these promises except one. He did tell Mr. de Leval when the trial was coming on. He never made any report of the progress of the trial, although it took two days. He never disclosed what the sentence was. He never informed the only powerful friends of his unhappy client that she was to be executed unless outside in‑tervention came. And when Mr. de Leval tried to find him he had disappeared.

# CHAPTER 9

# Trial in Secret

The conspirators had thus succeeded in drawing an impenetrable veil across their wicked purposes.

Practically the only accounts of the trial are those printed in the German newspapers a fortnight after the execution. These tell us that the court-martial was held in the Court of the Brussels Senate- House. The judges are not named. The principal person accused (says the *Hamburger Fremdenblatt*, which in the true German way assesses titles higher than all personal characteristics) was Prince Reginald de Croy, of Belignies, but he had not been found. The Princess Maria, his wife, stood, however, in the dock with Edith Cavell beside her.

Miss Cavell was in the nurse's uniform in which she had been arrested. The white cap covering the back of the head and disclosing the neat dark waved hair beginning to go grey at the sides, was tied beneath the chin with a starched bow. The stiff collar surmounted the white apron. On the nurse's arm was the red cross of her merciful calling. Her clear eyes looked out on a group of enemies. Overfed officers, with thick necks and coarse eyes, faced her from the judge's bench. Soldiers with fixed bayonets stood between the prisoners.

Although she knew her danger, Nurse Cavell did not flinch before her accusers. There was nothing defiant in her look. It was too serene for anger. But the judges must have noted the weakness of the woman they were condemning. She was fragile almost to delicacy. Two months of prison had made her complexion ashy white. She looked about the court with curiosity, and even in this supreme hour had time for a compassionate smile for those who were sharing her peril.

The German papers give us an outline of the prosecution "case.", They allege that Miss Cavell and Prince Reginald de Croy were the two principals in a widespread espionage organisation. Aided by the

French Countess of Belleville, they had assisted young Belgian, French, and British soldiers to escape from Belgium. The refugees were taken by different routes to Brussels, hidden in Miss Cavell's hospital or in a convent, and conducted by night in tramcars out of Brussels, and then by guides to loosely guarded points along the Dutch frontier.

When this statement was ended, Miss Cavell was asked to plead. In a low, gentle voice, contrasting with the harsh accents of her accusers, she replied that she believed she had served her country, and if that was wrong she was willing to take the blame. The lips of some of her fellow-prisoners quivered as they heard these brave words.

Fearlessly, and in quiet, firm tones, Miss Cavell went on to disclose facts which provided chapter and verse for her "crime." The questions were put in German, then translated by an interpreter into French, which Miss Cavell of course knew well. "She spoke without trembling and showed a clear mind," an eye-witness afterwards told Mr. de Leval. "Often she added some greater precision to her previous depositions."

The Military Prosecutor asked her why she had helped these soldiers to go to England. "If I had not done so they would have been shot," she answered. "I thought I was only doing my duty in saving their lives."

"That may be very true as regards English soldiers," responded the prosecutor, "Why did you help young Belgians to cross the frontier when they would have been perfectly safe in staying here?"

The answer to this question is not recorded. "In helping Belgians I help my own country" must have been the thought that rose to her lips.

Other prisoners were asked what they had to say, and among them, M. Philippe Bancq, a Belgian architect, made a memorable plea, fit to put beside Nurse Cavell's.

"I helped young Belgians to escape to join the army," he said. "As a good Belgian patriot I am ready to lay down my life for my country." Bancq has since been shot.

The prosecution asked for the death sentence to be passed upon Miss Cavell and eight other prisoners. But "the Judges did not seem to agree." Nurse Cavell's heroism appeared to have made some impression on her enemy's hearts.

Sentence was postponed. It seemed as though mercy might prevail.

# CHAPTER 10

# Fighting for Life

Between the trial and the sentence some sinister influence intervened. It is a secret of the Germans what that influence was. But we cannot follow the incidents of the last day of Edith Cavell's life without becoming aware that a design had been conceived in some brain to hurry on the last penalty before there was time for a reprieve.

Mr. de Leval had heard privately on the evening before (Sunday, October 10th) that the trial was over, and that the death sentence had been demanded. The trial had ended on Friday, but Mr. Kirschen, the lawyer, did not report to Mr. de Leval as he had promised. Neither on Saturday nor Sunday could Mr. Kirschen be found, and he disappears altogether from view after the trial. After fruitless inquiries on Sunday night, Mr. de Leval went to see Baron de Lancken, the German Political Minister. Late at night he succeeded in finding a subordinate, Mr. Conrad, but could obtain no information.

On the Monday morning Mr. de Leval again saw Conrad, who assured him that judgment would not be passed for a day or two, and that the American Legation would be informed as soon as this took place. No word came from Conrad all day, and none from Kirschen. The lawyer was "out till afternoon" Mr. de Leval was told when he called at the house.

On this crucial day Mr. Brand Whitlock, the American Minister, was ill in bed. But he was working hard to save Miss Cavell's life. With Mr. Hugh Gibson, Secretary of the Embassy, he prepared a letter to Baron Von der Lancken pointing out that Miss Cavell had spent her life in alleviating the sufferings of others, had bestowed her care as freely on the German soldiers as on others. "Her career as a servant of humanity," he wrote, "is such as to inspire every pity, to call for every pardon." And with his own hand the Minister wrote this touching appeal:—

> My dear Baron,—I am too ill to present my request to you
> in person, but I appeal to your generosity of heart to support
> it and save this unfortunate woman from death. Have pity on
> her!

Throughout the day the Legation made repeated inquiries of the
German authorities to know if sentence had been passed. The last was
at twenty minutes past six. Mr. Conrad then stated that sentence had
not been pronounced, and renewed his promise to let the Legation
know as soon as there was anything to tell.

At five o'clock that same afternoon the death sentence had been
passed in secret. The execution was fixed for the same night.

Three hours later the American Legation learned privately of the
deception. Mr. Gibson found the Spanish Ambassador, the Marquis de
Villalobar, and went with him to Baron Von der Lancken's house. The
Baron was "out" as the advocate had been in the morning. Neither
was any member of his staff at home. An urgent message was sent after
the Baron. He returned with two of his staff at a little after ten. The
execution was to take place at two next morning.

Lancken at first refused to believe that the death sentence had
been passed. Even if it had the execution would not be that night,
and "nothing could be done until next morning." But the two diplo-
matists refused to be put off. They compelled the Baron to make inquiries, and when he was obliged reluctantly to admit the truth, they
urged him to appeal to the Military Governor, Von Bissing.

At eleven o'clock Von der Lancken came back from seeing Von
Bissing. He brought a refusal. The Governor-General had acted "after
mature deliberation" and refused to listen to any plea of clemency. For
an hour longer the two devoted ministers pleaded for the woman's
life. It was in vain. There was no appeal. "Even the Emperor could
not intervene." Edith Cavell was doomed. At midnight her friends
departed in despair.

# CHAPTER 11

# The Last Scene

The most beautiful moments in Edith Cavell's life were those which preceded her martyrdom. At eleven o'clock the British chaplain in Brussels, the Rev. H. S. T. Gahan, was admitted to the cell in which she had spent the past ten weeks.

He found her calm and resigned. She told him that she wished all her friends to know that she gave her life willingly for her country. And then she used these imperishable words:—

I have no fear nor shrinking. I have seen death so often that it is not strange or fearful to me.

I thank God for this ten weeks' quiet before the end. Life has always been hurried and full of difficulty. This time of rest has been a great mercy.

They have all been very kind to me here. But this I would say, standing as I do in view of God and eternity, I realise that patriotism is not enough. I must have no hatred or bitterness to anyone.

After this the chaplain administered the Holy Communion. The clergyman repeated the words of *Abide with me*. She joined in at the words:

*Hold Thou Thy cross before my closing eyes;*
*Shine through the gloom, and point me to the skies;*
*Heaven's morning breaks, and earth's vain shadows flee.*
*In life, in death, O Lord, abide with me.*

At two o'clock in the morning they led her out with bandaged eyes to the place of execution. The firing party stood ready with loaded rifles. At this last moment her physical strength was not a match

38

for her heroic spirit. She fell in a swoon. The officer in charge of the soldiers stepped forward and shot her as she lay unconscious.

Before the day dawned her body was laid to rest in the land occupied by her enemies, whom with her last breath she forgave.

# Chapter 12

# Edith Cavell's Message

The circumstances of Edith Cavell's death became known in England on Trafalgar Day. The news reached the public through the newspapers the following morning. No one who was in London that day will ever forget the sense of horror that ran through the land. From early morning a dense crowd of people thronged round the only tangible symbol of her martyrdom, a wreath of laurels placed among those of the sailors who died for England. The armless Nelson looked down from his column upon the memorial of a weak woman who had borne witness to his immortal message. The seaman and officers who had died in the long-drawn-out Trafalgar, welcomed her, as it seemed, to their company. And in the mist and rain of a London October day the true spirit of England leaped again to life.

"This will settle the matter, once for all, about recruiting in Great Britain," said the Bishop of London. "There will be no need now of compulsion." All day men competed in their eagerness to join the Army. Continual recruiting meetings were held round the base of Nelson's monument. In Nurse Cavell's native village every eligible man joined the Forces next day. A tide of enthusiasm set in which has not yet waned.

Consternation and horror expressed themselves in every part of the world. The *Staats Zeitung*, the Germans' newspaper in New York which defended the sinking of the *Lusitania*, disowned the crime. "This is savagery," said neutral Holland. "The killing of Miss Cavell will be more expensive than the loss of many regiments," said a great American journal. "The peace of the future would be incomplete and precarious," wrote the Paris *Figaro*, "if crimes like these escaped the justice of peoples." The King and Parliament gave voice to England's sentiment.

Yet the Germans were so little conscious of what they had done that they made the deed blacker by excuses. "We hope it will serve as a warning to the Belgians," wrote the Berlin official paper, the *Vossische Zeitung*. "I know of no law in the world which makes distinction between the sexes," said Herr Zimmermann, the Kaiser's Under-Secretary for Foreign Affairs. And they filled the cup of their infamy by refusing to surrender Nurse Cavell's body to her friends.

It is fitting that there should be some personal memorial to this heroic life. One such, by the thoughtful initiative of Queen Alexandra, is to be provided in the shape of an Edith Cavell Nursing Home at the London Hospital where Miss Cavell was trained. The *Nursing Mirror*, for which she wrote her last article, urges the institution of a Cavell Cross for Heroism, a decoration for women only.

An Empire Day of Homage has been proposed. A great national memorial service has been held in St. Paul's Cathedral.

But the best memorial to Edith Cavell will be the determination of her fellow-citizens to put aside self in willing service to their country.

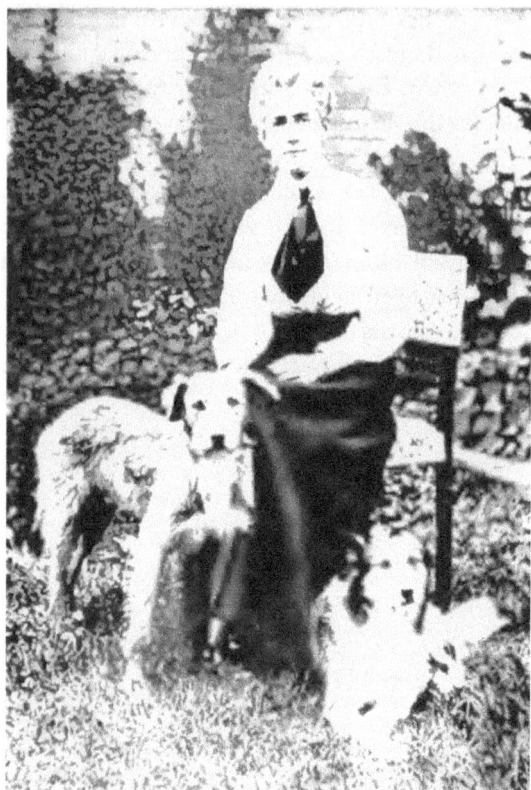

Nurse Cavell in her garden

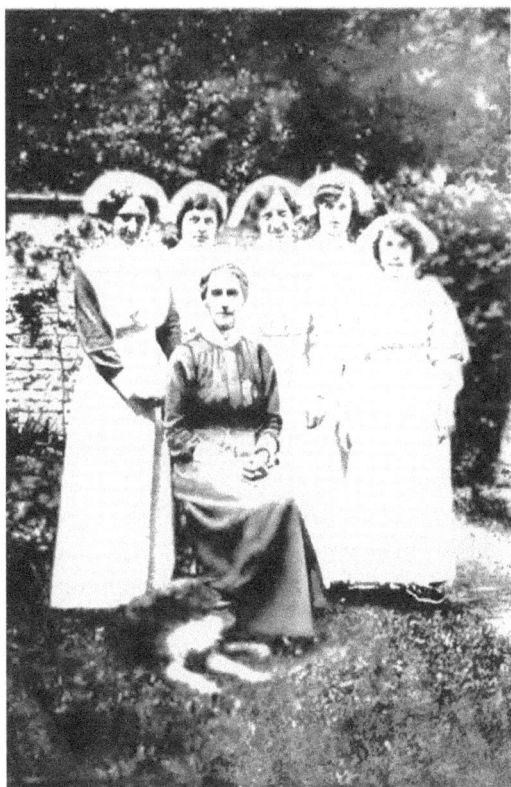

NURSE CAVELL,
FROM A PHOTOGRAPH TAKEN IN BRUSSELS.

# Appendix

## SIR EDWARD GREY'S SCATHING COMMENT

Sir Edward Grey to the American Ambassador in London.

Foreign Office, October 20th, 1915.

The Secretary of State for Foreign Affairs presents his compliments to the United States Ambassador, and has the honour to acknowledge the receipt of His Excellency's note of the 18th instant enclosing a copy of a despatch from the United States Minister at Brussels respecting the execution of Miss Edith Cavell at that place.

Sir E. Grey is confident that the news of the execution of this noble Englishwoman will be received with horror and disgust not only in the Allied States, but throughout the civilised world.

Miss Cavell was not even charged with espionage, and the fact that she had nursed numbers of wounded German soldiers might have been regarded as a complete reason in itself for treating her with leniency.

The attitude of the German authorities is, if possible, rendered worse by the discreditable efforts successfully made by the officials of the German Civil Administration at Brussels to conceal the fact that sentence had been passed and would be carried out immediately. These efforts were no doubt prompted by the determination to carry out the sentence before an appeal from the finding of the court-martial could be made to a higher authority, and show in the clearest manner that the German authorities concerned were well aware that the carrying out of the sentence was not warranted by any consideration.

Further comment on their proceedings would be superfluous.

In conclusion, Sir E. Grey would request Mr. Page to express

44

to Mr. Whitlock and the staff of the United States Legation at Brussels the grateful thanks of His Majesty's Government for their untiring efforts on Miss Cavell's behalf. He is fully satisfied that no stone was left unturned to secure for Miss Cavell a fair trial, and when sentence had been pronounced a mitigation thereof.

Sir E. Grey realises that Mr. Whitlock was placed in a very embarrassing position by the failure of the German authorities to inform him that the sentence had been passed and would be carried out at once. In order, therefore, to forestall any unjust criticism which might be made in this country he is publishing Mr. Whitlock's despatch to Mr. Page without delay.

## THE GERMAN OFFICIAL DEFENCE.

### Statement by Herr Zimmermann, German Under-Secretary of State for Foreign Affairs.

It is indeed hard that a woman has to be executed, but think what a State is to come to which is at war if it allows to pass unnoticed a crime against the safety of its armies because it is committed by women. No law book in the world, least of all those dealing with war regulations, makes such a differentiation, and the female sex has but one preference according to legal usage, namely, that women in a delicate condition may not be executed. Otherwise a man and woman are equal before the law, and only the degree of guilt makes a difference in the sentence for a crime and its consequences.

In the Cavell case all the circumstances are so clear and convincing that no court-martial in the world could have reached any other decision. For it concerns not the act of one single person, but rather a well-thought-out, world-wide conspiracy, which succeeded for nine months in rendering the most valuable service to the enemy, to the disadvantage of our army.

### SEVERITY THE ONLY WAY.

Countless British, Belgian and French soldiers are now again fighting in the Allies' ranks who owe their escape from Belgium to the activity of the band now sentenced, at the head of which stood Miss Cavell.

With such a situation under the very eyes of the authorities only the utmost severity can bring relief, and a Government violates the most elementary duty towards its army that does not adopt the strictest measures. These duties in war are greater than any other.

All those convicted were fully cognisant of the significance of their actions. The court went into just this point with particular care, and acquitted several co-defendants because it believed a doubt existed regarding their knowledge of the penalties for their actions.

I admit, certainly, that the motive of those convicted was not unnoble, that they acted out of patriotism; but in war time one must be ready to seal one's love of Fatherland with one's blood.

### To Frighten the Others.

Once for all, the activity of our enemies has been stopped, and the sentence has been carried out to frighten those who might presume on their sex to take part in enterprises punishable with death. Should one recognise these presumptions it would open the door for the evil activities of women, who often are handier and cleverer in these things than the craftiest spy.

If the others are shown mercy it will be at the cost of our army, for it is to be feared that new attempts will be made to injure us if it is believed that escape without punishment is possible or with the risk of only a light sentence.

Only pity for the guilty can lead to a commutation. It will not be an admission that the executed sentence was too severe, for this, harsh as it may sound, was absolutely just, and could not appear otherwise to an independent judge.

It is asserted that the soldiers told off to carry out the execution refused at first to shoot, and finally fired so faultily that an officer had to kill the accused with his revolver.

No word of this is true. I have an official report of the execution, in which it is established that it took place entirely in accordance with the established regulations, and that death occurred immediately after the first volley, as the physician present attests.

# With Edith Cavell in Belgium

Jacqueline Van Til

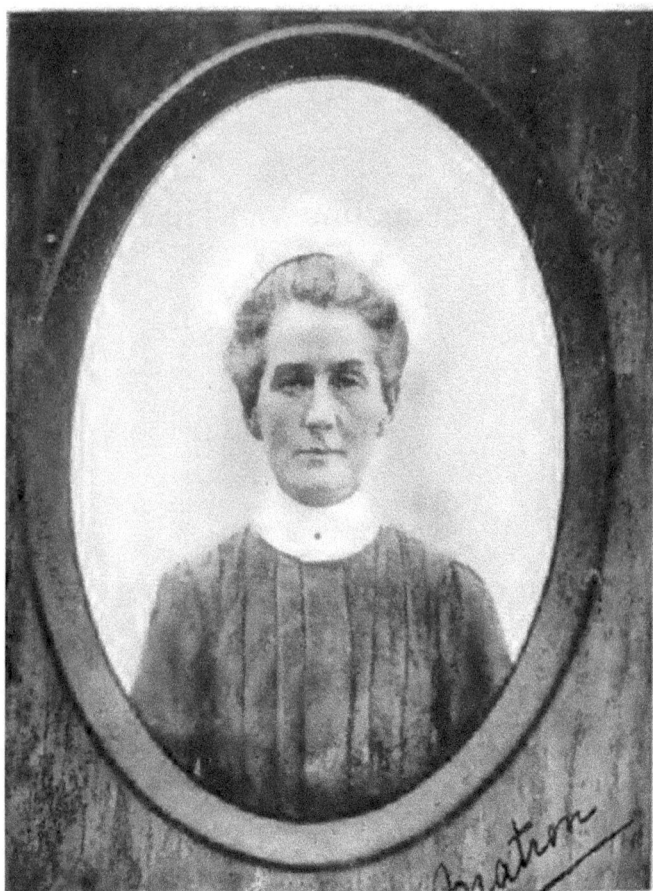

Nurse Edith Cavell

# Contents

... HERE AND THERE, A WHISPERED WORD,
EVEN THOUGH UTTERED WITHOUT BAD INTENTION,
HAS MANY TIMES RUINED THE GOOD NAME,
THE REPUTATION
AND EVEN THE LIFE OF SOMEBODY.

EDITH CAVELL.

# Introduction

When, a year ago, I came to the United States, I was often forced to speak in broken English about the five wonderful years which I spent in Brussels under the same roof with England's martyred nurse, Edith Cavell.

Many persons seemed to be interested in what I had to say; among them was a friend, Mr. José de Muro, who advised me to write for the American people what I knew of Miss Cavell's life while with her in Belgium.

I tried, but my slight knowledge of the English language made my task a very difficult one.

I am aware that many pages of this humble narrative are not of great literary merit. But I do claim that every word of it is true.

Jacqueline Van Til,<br>Former Trained Nurse of<br>Edith Cavell, Brussels.

White Plains, April 27, 1921.

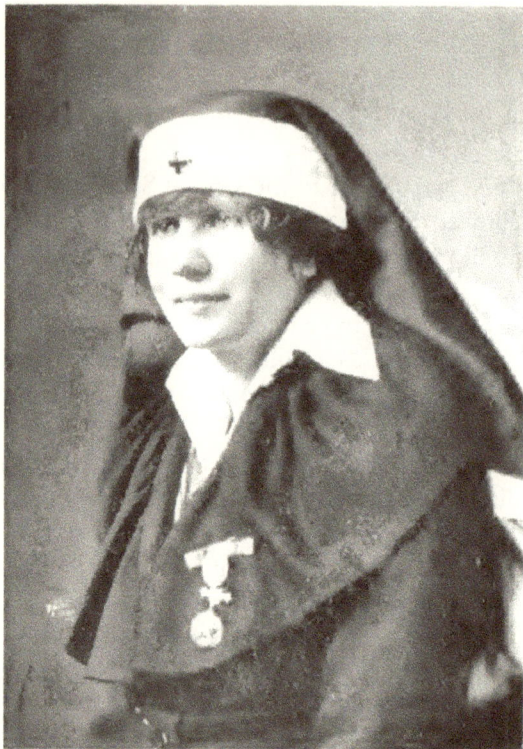

JACQUELINE VAN TIL, R. N.

CHAPTER 1

# Before the War

It was in the month of December, 1910, that a friend and I were going, for the first time, to the Edith Cavell Clinique, called *L'école Belge pour les Infirmières Diplomées*, in Brussels.

The weather was very cold that evening, when we rang the bell at what was to be our future home, and we were not sorry to have reached a place of shelter. A well-dressed maid opened the door, and conducted us to the room where Miss Edith Cavell was at work. This was the first time we had met. She made a deep impression on us. I distinctly remember that we felt quite uneasy at her gaze, for she impressed us as being very tall and distinguished. At that time of her life, she was about forty years of age. Her eyes were blue; they would soften while she talked to us, but would become very stern and dark, when the little maid that was there dared to interrupt us.

Her mouth was expressive, the lines around it were hard, both lips were extremely thin,—a trait that denoted strength of will and firmness of character. Her hair, a dark blonde, with silver strands at the temples, was neatly coiled on the back of her head. Her voice was clear and precise, and she spoke the French language with a charming English accent. Her movements were simple, and her little hand felt very soft when she grasped ours to welcome us to her home. She conducted us to our rooms and showed us the places where the nurses were allowed to go, and where they could amuse themselves with music or with needlework.

Our *clinique* was not very large; and from the outside looked rather poor and inadequate. It was composed of four ordinary houses, two of them for the patients and two for the nurses and the servants. The numbers of the latter were 149 and 147, and those of the former 145 and 143. They were situated in the *rue de la Culture*, a street that

55

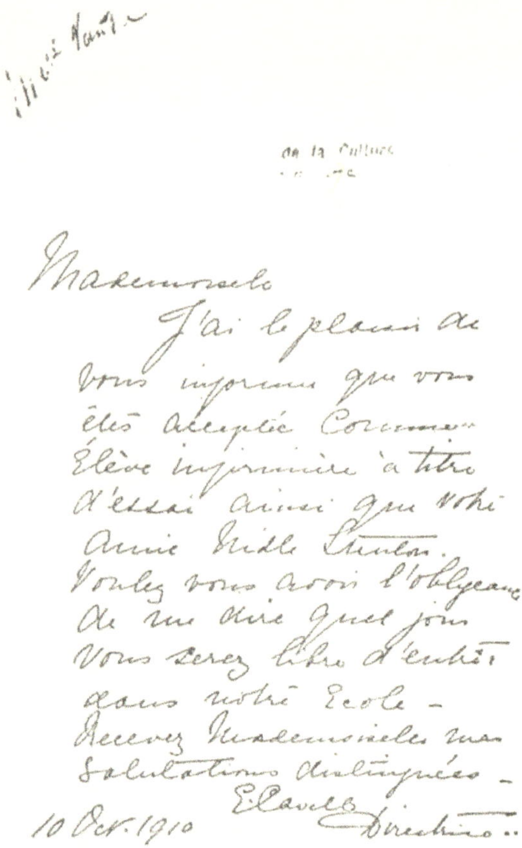

*[handwritten letter in French]*

de la Culture

Mademoiselle

J'ai le plaisir de
vous informer que vous
êtes acceptée comme
Élève infirmière à titre
d'essai ainsi que votre
amie Miss Stenton.
Voulez vous avoir l'obligeance
de me dire quel jour
vous serez libre d'entrer
dans notre École —
Recevez Mademoiselle mes
Salutations distinguées —

E. Cavell
Directrice

10 Oct. 1910

ORIGINAL LETTER OF EDITH CAVELL,
WHICH I RECEIVED FROM HER IN 1910.

149, Rue de la Culture,
Brussels,
Telephone 9559.

*Mademoiselle:*

I have the pleasure of informing you that you are accepted as a
pupil nurse on probation as well as your friend, Miss Stenton.
Will you have the kindness to inform me on what day you will
be free to enter our school?

Pray accept, *Mademoiselle*, my respectful salutations.

E. Cavell,
*Directrice*

10th October, 1910.

formed part of a suburb of Brussels named "Ixelles," and were about an hour's walk from that city.

Because those four houses were much too small to contain all the nurses, Miss Cavell had decided to lodge some of the latter in another house at No. 140, in the same street, where she rented ten rooms for the private nurses, the public-health nurses, and nurses who worked outside the little *clinique*.

The patients' rooms were well furnished and were painted white. The small operating-room was very well equipped indeed. Many patients were quite thankful to go to the small *clinique*, which was sometimes called "The English Nursing Home," in the *rue de la Culture*.

In these houses we had room for thirty patients and each one had his own doctor. These were all private cases, but sometimes we nursed some poor chronic cases from the community, though, as a rule, we had only well-paying patients.

The nurses were obliged to be trained in different hospitals, as the *clinique* was too small to give them a good training. These nurses were, for the first year, under Miss Edith Cavell's special care, and they were given lectures and received practical training from fourteen physicians. The second year, she sent them to the different hospitals which she had founded during the time she was there; and, after three years of training elsewhere, they came back to her own hospital, where she perfected them in the science of nursing the sick.

Until now, there were very few Belgian girls at the *clinique*, as our Belgian people were not yet able to understand the meaning of Nurse-work. Most of us were strangers from different countries,— from Germany as well as from France and England; and all of us had to speak French when on duty. We were sixty in all, when my friend and I came here, in 1910, and I never shall forget how comical this little place seemed, filled as it was with the loud laughter and songs of the nurses, each in her own tongue.

Miss Cavell never objected to various nationalities, all she required of us was obedience to her orders as well as to those of her assistant supervisors. This we well knew, and in all the years that I served her, I never met with a nurse who dared to disobey.

During the first year, we stood in fear of her, for her remarks were oft-times severe and laconic. We never dared to come too late to table, knowing beforehand that we should encounter the stern reproach of her dark blue eyes, and the hard expression of her lips. How sorry I am, now, when I think of those moments during which we nurses

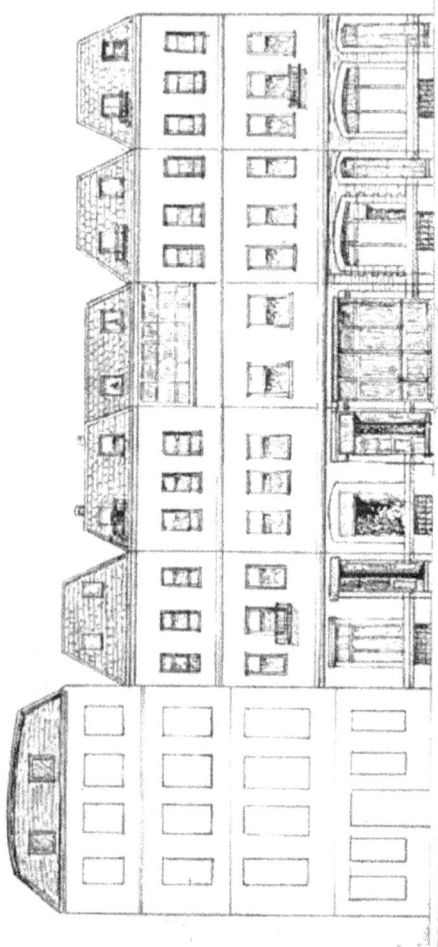

CLINIQUE.

1907 — 1915

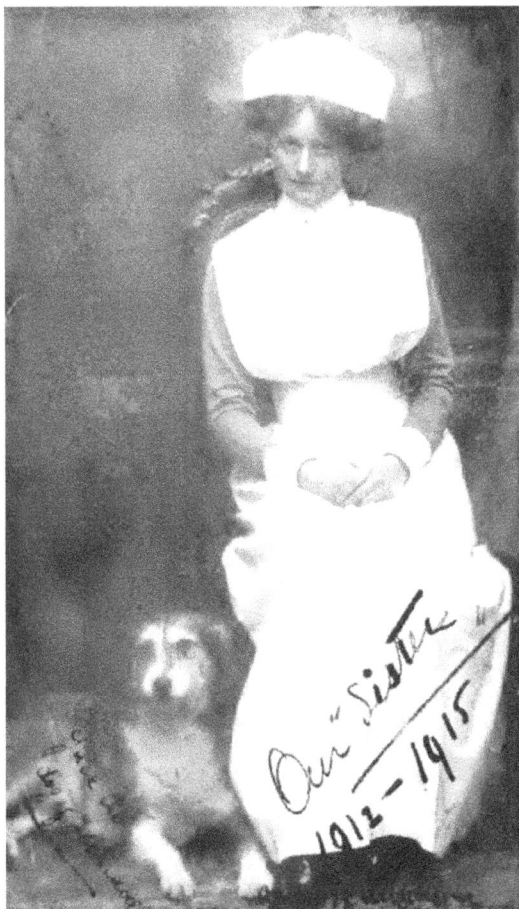

SISTER WILKINS AND JACK,
MISS CAVELL'S SHEPHERD DOG

used to talk together about her and criticise her as being too severe! We little understood at that time, that her task was so difficult; that she was all alone in looking after the organization and management of everything she had founded.

When, in the year 1907, she came to Brussels, as a private nurse to the Graux family. Dr. DePage, one of our great surgeons, noticed the wonderful gifts of this English nurse. This doctor had encountered many difficulties in his work, on account of not having been properly assisted in nursing. He wished to start real trained nursing for the sick in Belgium, as it existed already in England and Holland. He talked the matter over with some rich persons in his city, and with Miss Cavell's friends, the Graux family. A committee was formed, and they offered Miss Cavell the position of superintendent of a home where young girls could be trained as nurses.

For this purpose they rented four houses in the *rue de la Culture*, and had them arranged into a small *clinique*. Some publicity was given to the undertaking, and many posters were affixed to the walls of the houses of Brussels, with the words: "*Young Girls Wanted*," etc., written in large red letters.

When Miss Edith Cavell entered upon her new undertaking, in October, 1907, she had only four nurses, and two supervisors. The latter were English and did not know a word of French. Moreover, of these four nurses, three were Swiss girls, and the fourth was a Belgian girl, the only one of that nationality there.

Speaking to me on this subject, Miss Cavell said that the beginning had been very trying in the small *clinique*. The doctors, she added, had been too familiar with the nurses, and the English rules of her hospital were not always followed.

Her will was strong, however, and she fought bravely against the lack of funds on the one hand, and the insincerity and narrow-mindedness of individuals on the other, but, in spite of these obstacles, she came off victorious.

After one year's experience of trained nursing, in her establishment in the *rue de la Culture*, the doctors began to value her abilities, and to treat the nurses with more respect.

It was at this time that, at the large Hospital of St. Gilles, under Dr. DePage, the nuns were dismissed, and Miss Cavell was installed in their place. The same change occurred in Dr. Meyer's sanatorium, where she laid down the first rules for the training of nurses, and, when I came, in 1910, she was already at the head of several hospitals in Brussels, together with the Tuberculosis Hospital at Buysinghen, a little village in Wallonie, Belgium.

The same year, with only three workers, she placed nurses in the public-schools. In 1915 there were twelve of them. She also sent trained nurses out on private cases.

Her task was very hard indeed, for the members of the committee had lost some interest in the small *clinique*, and financial help was lacking; so that Miss Cavell had to depend entirely upon herself for the management of everything; for the young nurses, whom she was striving to convert into useful help, were thoughtlessly amusing themselves, while she was worrying over the lack of funds and the many other difficulties she had to encounter in her task.

In the years 1910 and 1911 very few changes occurred. I attended the classes for trained nurses, and like the other nurses I was sent to the different hospitals. Miss Cavell, whom we were in the habit of calling *Madame*, used to walk, three times a day, to and from the different places where she sent her nurses, and she was invariably followed there by her two dogs, Jack and Don. I can still imagine I see her, walking along, with a slight stoop, accompanied by one of the patients, smiling pleasantly at the children whom she met along her way.

All the patients were fond of her, and in the whole *clinique*, there was not a soul who could give more comfort to a suffering patient than she, and though she had many duties to fulfil, yet she always found time to sit at the bedside of pain and sorrow, where she would minister to the sick, and inwardly pray for the sufferer's soul.

Every night, at eight o'clock, we were required to attend the class-room, where it was her habit to instruct us in everything relating to the different diseases. She was indefatigable in teaching us, and never spared herself in anything that required labour. When I look back, now, to that time, I cannot help but feel ashamed of myself to think that I, sometimes, could scarcely keep awake during the lecture, and when she would say to me, in a soft voice, "Mile. Van Til, won't you please sit next to me? I don't think that you can follow the lecture very well," I could not keep from showing my chagrin. During my first year with her she seemed not to take much notice of me, but often the nurses would be called to her office to be admonished for loud laughter, and also advised to be careful of their manners.

In 1912 I was taken ill, and was transferred to a small room on the second floor, where Miss Cavell personally took care of me. I still can feel the touch of her soft white hand, gently gliding over my hair, her

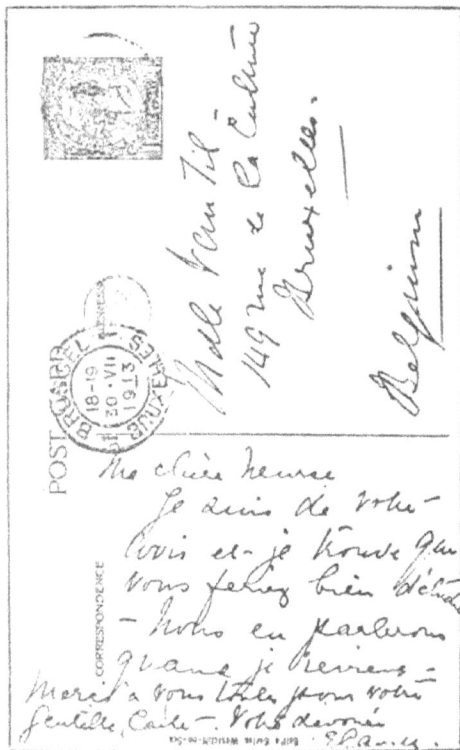

POSTCARD FROM EDITH CAVELL WHILE SHE
WAS IN ENGLAND

My dear Nurse:

I think you are right to go on with your
studies. We will talk about it, when I come
back. Thanks very much for your nice card.

Yours truly,

E. Cavell.

deep blue eyes peering into my fever-flushed face.

She nursed me through it all, and when I was able to sit up, she would sit by my side and assure me that the good Lord had been with me all the while. She moreover told me that from that time on she would be like a mother to me. I shall ever recall those moments with gratitude and emotion, so clear and strong is their image engraved in my soul!

As I did not look strong upon leaving the sickbed, *Madame* sent me to England to recuperate at her sister's home in Henley-on-Thames. The husband of the latter was a Dr. Wainright. They lived in a charming house called "Upton Lodge." Here I met her dear old mother, and her other sister, Florence, who was a superintendent in a London Hospital. While I was stopping here I learned that Miss Cavell was born in 1865, in the vicinity of Norwich, and that her father had been a clergyman, who, when he died, left his wife in the care of his daughter Florence. Miss Cavell had a brother whom I did not see; but, while there, I met many of her friends, who belonged to some of the best families of England.

After remaining at her sister's home for a few weeks, I was sufficiently recovered to be able to return to the small *clinique* in Belgium, and continue my work.

Here a few changes had occurred, during my absence in England. The committee was now being assisted by a Mr. Goldsmith, a wealthy banker, who offered to furnish money for a new Nurses' School to be built in the *Rue de la Bruxelles*. I remember, one evening, having been shown the plans by *Madame*, herself, and I noticed how happy she was about it. She determined to look after all the plans. She succeeded so well that the new Nurses' Building was started in 1913. This same year I worked permanently with her in the *clinique*, while I learned more and more about her great ability, and when she went to her home in England, to spend her vacation with her family, I was left in charge of a section of the place.

When she returned from England, in August, 1913, she had with her a young girl of fifteen, named Pauline Randell, whom she had found abandoned by her parents.

*Madame* decided to become a god-mother to the girl, and employed her as a general help around the house. From that time on, 'Madame, Pauline, and Jack, the shepherd dog, could be seen strolling together every day to the different hospitals where some of her nurses were employed.

We nurses did not take kindly to Pauline, and we detested Jack. Her other dog, Don, had been stolen from her in 1911, to our great delight; for he annoyed us with his pranks; but Jack became fiercer than Don had been, and though he was a true and faithful dog, yet he would try to bite everyone who dared to look at his mistress. As regards Pauline, our dislike for her was from another cause. She was not a wicked girl, but she was haughty with us, and of a jealous disposition, and had a way of reporting us to her mistress for the slightest error in our duties. Perhaps it is unkind of me to write this, and also unkind in us not to have been more generous and fair towards her and the dog; because they both rendered great assistance to their mistress in this house of many troubles.

This same year, Madame Marie DePage, wife of Dr. DePage, began to take more interest in the work of nursing than she had hitherto done; she now assisted *Madame* in the administration of the hospital, and was very kind to us. Although her character was quite the opposite of that of *Madame*, yet they agreed, and, after a short time, they became close friends. Here I cannot help thinking how strange it seems to me that both these high-souled women died for their country, each of them in such a sad way.

In the beginning of the year 1914 there was an Armenian boy, named "Jose," who had been educated in Belgium, and of whom *Madame* took great care. This boy had shown himself to be honest and faithful, and he showed such a good character that she took him into her service, where he performed special duties allotted to him by his mistress. I make particular mention of this boy, in this place, because he afterward became well known to us, and played a worthy role in the sad drama of Miss Edith Cavell; and, like so many others who served in the same cause, he, too, has been forgotten.

As usual, at the end of July, of the same year, *Madame* took her vacation in England with Pauline, leaving a supervisor named Miss Wilkins in charge of the *clinique*. The very day after she left, I went to Lille, to pay a visit to some friends of mine there, little dreaming that a great war was impending, and menacing the existence of my country and my own happy and peaceful life. When I reached the French border I was forced to remain for the whole night at the small station of Quévy. Everybody was talking about Germany, but I did not pay much attention to it. I reached Lille the next day, and there, too, everyone seemed very much upset. I decided that it would be best for me to return to Brussels. I arrived there on the fourth of August and went straight to the *rue de la Culture*, where I found that Miss Cavell and Pauline had just come back from England.

*Madame* appeared very calm, as she usually was, and said to me that she thought it best for her to stay with her nurses, now that their country seemed to be in danger. In spite of her calmness, however, many of her nurses left, first the German and then the Dutch girls, reducing greatly the personnel of the already small *clinique*.

## Chapter 2

# Outbreak of War

Those were very troublesome days, just before the war was declared. *Madame* had a hard time trying to keep the young nurses together, and endeavoured to calm them by assuring them that it would probably not occur, or that, at all events, it would not last long. Her efforts were all lost, however, for when on the very next day, the fifth of August, 1914, the Belgian Army officers, in their war automobiles, drove up and down the streets to call up recruits for the army, all our nurses were seized with a panic. Yet it was *Madame* who told us to think of our patients, and to remain and do our duty toward them. She succeeded in calming us, and did not seem very anxious, for she herself was at that time convinced that the Germans would never reach Brussels.

We got most of the beds of our *clinique* ready to receive wounded Belgian soldiers. Nearly all the patients had left—many of them in great haste—because of their fear of the Germans; and like all the rich, they went to the sea-shore, thinking that the Prussians would never dare to come there.

All the wealthy men of Brussels who did not desire to join the army, had their homes made ready for the wounded. We called these little hospitals "ambulances." There were more than twelve hundred of these in existence when the Germans finally arrived.

Our *clinique*, as I have mentioned above, was situated in a suburb of the city, and by this time no patients remained, so that *Madame* sent some of her nurses, myself included, to a large ambulance base in the city. A few days before this, the King and Queen had left for Antwerp. The royal consort had previously given up her beautiful palace to be used as an ambulance station, and Marie DePage had been received there by Her Majesty as its superintendent.

Dr. LeBoeuf, the Queen's private physician, assisted Madame De-Page, and remained attached to this ambulance base throughout the war.

In those days, when we first heard the German cannons booming over the frontier, and when their soldiers seemed, each moment, to be coming nearer and nearer—we had not, as yet, known what war really was—everything so peaceful and calm in our *clinique* to which we returned every night from the city to rest.

In the St. Jean's Ambulance, where I worked, there was only one Belgian patient, so far, and he had never seen a German. He was a bicyclist that had been sent to Liége, but never reached there, having fallen from his wheel and broken his left arm. Being the only wounded soldier we had in our place we made much of him, and you can imagine what a glorious time he had!

Things were not yet so very sad in Brussels; the streets were lively and crowded with recruits for the army, and our little "*Jass*," [1] laughing and hopeful, was starting for the German border. Even at the railroad stations we met with smiling faces, and no one seemed to realize the gravity of the event. What did we know, at that time, about war and cannons? But, alas, when the Germans finally did enter Brussels, we could hardly believe our eyes!

Sorrow, now, took the place of gaiety on those faces which but a short while before had been so full of sunshine and levity. Had it not been for our *burgomaster*, the brave Mr. Max, many terrible events might have occurred.

Our misfortunes had already begun, when we heard the sound of the German cannon close to the Belgian capital, just as the last trains had left it for the sea-shore.

We, now, were beginning to feel very uneasy. During the evenings, the excitement in the streets was profound, and the windows of the German business houses and stores were broken by angry Belgian citizens, who would become exasperated upon hearing anyone speak with a foreign accent, and immediately try to knock the strangers down.

The excitement was considerably increased when some Belgians came with the news that Louvain, that proud and famous old Flemish town, was burning, though the daily paper, *Le Soir*, one of the few that were still issued, had not mentioned the disaster at all—probably with

---

1. "*Jass*" is the Flemish term for the Belgian soldier, like the word "*Toilu*" is for the French.—Author's note.

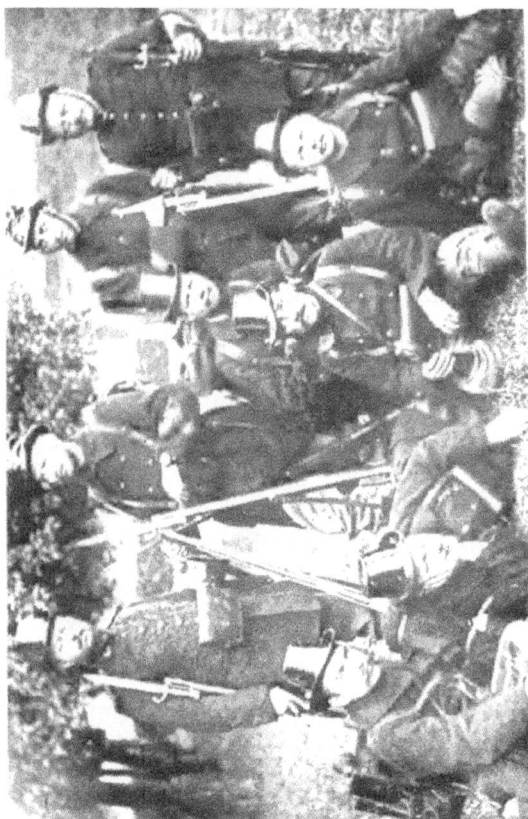

BELGIAN CIVIL-SOLDIERS IN PRE–WAR UNIFORMS

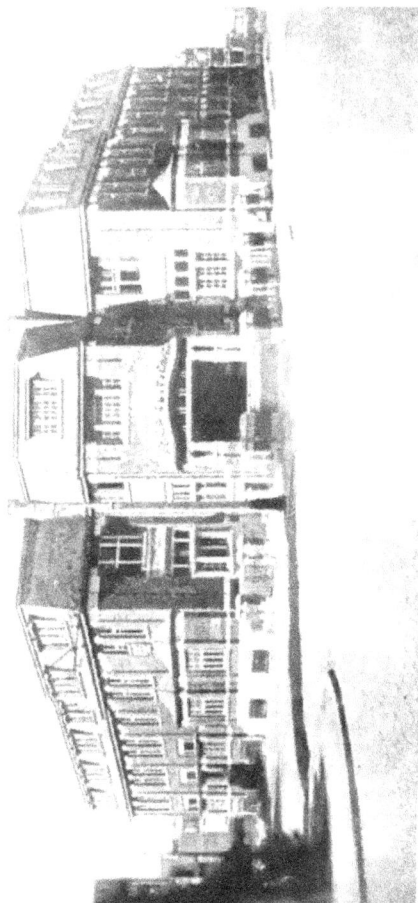

THE EDITH CAVELL CLINIQUE

the thoughtful intention of keeping the people quiet. But when the first refugees from Tervueren, a small village about five miles from the Belgian capital, arrived and informed us of all the horrors committed by the Germans in Louvain, we were utterly horrified.

I shall never forget the evening before the Prussians entered Brussels, when some of the nurses and I went up to the roof of our *clinique* and saw the sky, toward the East and the North-East, all a fiery red with glaring rockets and exploding shells, and accompanied by enormous clouds of thick, black smoke, which came rolling ominously in our direction. It was an awe-inspiring sight, and Its effect was greatly increased by the terrific din of the ever-booming cannon, the concussion of which was so intense that many window-panes were broken around us.

Many persons fled in great haste from Brussels, abandoning their former happy homes to the mercy of the cruel invaders.

All our nurses were crying and trembling with fear. I, too, was frightened. *Madame* found me sitting on the landing of the stairs, weeping bitterly. She peered into my upturned face, with that calm powerful gaze of hers, with something mild, yet full of firm reproach in it, and bade me not to give way to my feelings, that my life no longer belonged to myself alone, but also to my duty as a nurse. And she finally succeeded in calming me, as she did the other nurses; for, whenever there was an occasion for her to use persuasion, she always knew the proper thing to say to her nurses.

So, the very next day, I went as usual to the Ambulance Station where I had been detailed to work. We had nothing to do there, however, for the solitary Belgian soldier-patient of whom we had to take care had nearly recovered from his broken arm. The time seemed to drag on us; from nine o'clock until two, the hours seemed to us to creep very slowly along.

Then, all at once, our janitress, a very stout woman, suddenly ran into the hall, shouting excitedly in French: "*Les Boches sont là! Les Boches sont là!*"[2] We were all thrown into a state of confusion, and seemed spell-bound, the medical staff as well as the nurses. One of the doctors burst out crying, some of the nurses fainted. I was trembling all over with excitement, and I thought that the best thing for me to do was to go outdoors and get some fresh air. Immediately I, together with my friend, Miss Stenton, went out into the street, where thousands of citizens, with blanched faces, were standing mournfully around.

2. Meaning, "The Huns are coming!"—Author's note.

We followed some of the crowd to the street corner, but when we reached the place we could not hear a word that was said. We then went to the barracks situated in the suburbs, to get some information from the guardians there, but not a soul was to be seen. The large buildings were quite deserted. This made things look sad, indeed, to us; and to add to our sorrow, nature itself appeared to be laughing at our misfortunes, and seemed to conspire against us with the enemies; for the golden sun was pouring its brilliant light over the long columns of the German troops that were steadily advancing toward us. My friend and I both sat upon a rail fence by the roadside to view the rows upon rows of oncoming soldiers. They were approaching from four sides, and they looked like monster snakes with sinuous, winding bodies issuing from between the tall grass on either side of the road.

In spite of our fear and hatred of these foes, we could not help being fascinated at the sight of this great army, the pick of the German troops, as they passed in front of us, looking rosy-faced and well-fed, though somewhat awkward, with their heads held stiff, and the proud, triumphant smile of the conqueror on their faces. They advanced in rows of eight men each and between their ranks some poor Belgian prisoners were walking painfully along in their bare feet. This was a piteous sight indeed for us to view, and at it, our hatred for our country's foes grew suddenly strong, and impelled us to remain where we were, and gaze our fill. When we had seen enough we found a means of following a section of these troops to the *Grande Place de Brussels*, or the principal square. Here Mr. Max, our brave *burgomaster*, was awaiting the arrival of the Germans.

Everyone was now quiet in the street. The shop-windows were all tightly closed; the curtains in all the houses were lowered, and all this, by order of our prudent *burgomaster*, who, the evening before, had announced that all individuals who did not follow these rules would not be considered as true Belgians. This notice was posted on all the walls of Brussels.

It was here, in *La Grande Place* of the Capital of Belgium, that the well-beloved *burgomaster* received the German Commander, a tall, heavily built man, who demanded the surrender of the city. Accordingly, Mr. Max, standing upright, his head erect and his face deathly pale, decorously handed the keys of the city, the emblem of its liberty, to the smiling and bowing conqueror before him. I was not close enough to see his eyes, but I am certain that persons standing near him could not fail to notice the dignified gaze of our beloved *burgomaster*.

In the evening of the same eventful, weary day, several German papers placarded on the city walls, proclaimed to the inhabitants that the "Prussians were our masters." But, between two large notices, could be seen a smaller proclamation, printed in red ink, in French and in Flemish, which ran thus:

> We are Belgians! The only legal master we have is our rightful sovereign, King Albert. The present conquerors may have rules for their own people. We Have Ours!
>
> Signed:
>
> Max, *Burgomaster* of Brussels.

The very next day, he was sent away to Germany, as a prisoner, and he remained an exile there for the duration of the war.

This made a very sad impression on the hearts of our people, and caused the circling war-clouds to appear darker and darker around our beloved city.

As a consequence of the entry of the Prussians into Brussels, everything in our ambulance station was entirely changed, we now had many German soldiers to nurse, that had been wounded at Liége, Louvain, Tervueren and other places along the invader's line of march.

On the evening before, when *Madame* had called us together, to impress the idea upon us, that it was our duty, above all, to nurse all the wounded of whatever nation, under the influence of her powerful will, I did not dare to make known to her my profound disgust for my country's foes. So that I, together with the rest of the nurses, went, as was our custom, to the ambulance station, to aid in allaying the suffering of the injured patients; for some of the latter were badly wounded and also ill-clad.

Among our hospital supplies, we had much clothing that had been donated by wealthy patrons, but it was made for Belgian soldiers, who, as a rule, are small in stature and light of weight; so that when we had to put these under-sized garments on the tall, big, clumsy German patients, they were, of course, much too short and too tight, making the Prussians appear so ludicrous to us that, in spite of our sorrows, we could scarcely keep from laughing.

Here I shall have to relate what occurred to the solitary Belgian soldier that was still in our care. The next day after the Boches arrived, he remained hidden away in a small room in our building, and we, fearing that he would be caught by the enemy, determined upon helping him to escape. So, that night, we led him to the gardener's house, and there he managed to give the Huns the slip. I have never, since then, heard what became of him; though I have still the image of his large blue eyes with their childlike kindly expression, strongly engraved on my mind.

The days that followed these soul-stirring and painful events in our city were filled with trouble and sadness to the Belgian people. The arrival of the German troops, and the Proclamation of their commander completely changed our former conditions; from the free and happy people that we had been so shortly before, we were now reduced to the state of unhappy prisoners. The enemy soon made us feel their authority. Every day, there would occur many arrests of Belgian citizens, who had not followed the new laws of the invaders. The latter had already taken full possession of the city, and had installed themselves in the abandoned homes of those of the inhabitants that had fled to the seashore, or to England and Holland. All the military barracks, as well as all the public schools, and ambulance stations were crowded to the brim with German soldiers, who deliberately destroyed the stores of carefully sewn military clothing—the work of our brave Belgian women—that had been hastily abandoned by our retreating army.

The departure of our King and Queen made things seem all the sadder for us, since the details of it were so conflicting. When we thought that the Royal couple were still in Antwerp, they were actually running a thousand dangers on the sea, on their way to England.

Food and all the daily necessities of life had, by this time, become excessively expensive, and some of the most useful commodities were allowed to be taken only by the invaders; so that there was very little indeed left for us.

Two days afterward, the enormous army of the Germans (greatly increased by the continuous arrival of fresh troops from the Fatherland), was divided into two main fighting bodies, of which one division was sent to Antwerp, through Malines and Termond, both of which towns they ruthlessly destroyed, the other division was sent to France, by way of Waterloo, Mons, Namur, Charleroi, etc.

The cannon were booming night and day, and the horrid din of exploding shells was appalling. The forts of Antwerp fell, one after another, and it seemed to us that darkness and horror had chosen a dwelling place within our souls.

*Madame* alone, was as calm as ever. She continued tranquilly to direct us in all our duties.

So far, nothing was changed in our small *clinique*. The reason for this was that the suburb in which it was situated was somewhat remote from the German Headquarters, and that the enemy preferred to dwell in the city itself rather than in such an out-of-the-way place as was Ixelles; and therefore we had not yet been annoyed by their presence.

*Madame* went, every day, accompanied by Pauline and Jack, to the St. Gilles' Hospital, where some of her nurses were still working; she, also, went daily to the place where the building for the new Nurses' Training School had been started, which she could still visit without the least hindrance from the invaders.

Nevertheless, every night, she would call us together and seem to search into our inmost souls to see if we lacked courage; and she would endeavour to instil into us ideas of hope and fortitude. Up to the present time she had not shown much concern about the enemies' advance into our country. She did not speak much about them to us. Yet, she showed the loving tenderness of her womanly nature, by her constant solicitude for the welfare and care of the wounded.

As for myself, I still frequented the Ambulance Station, where, already, many of the enemies' wounded were to be found, some of them struggling in the throes of death. Many were mere lads, and many, fathers of families, people just like our own, but our enemies now, dying around us, and most of them labouring under the impression that they had conquered, and had reached their long cherished goal—"Paris!"

We cared for them, just the same as if they were our own wounded. But, when some of the least injured recovered sufficiently to be able to carry a gun, they were immediately sent to the front for the purpose, as we knew only too well, of killing our brothers and fathers. This was a cruel destiny for us, indeed, to be forced to help in nursing back to health these, our country's foes, only to assist them in gaining a victory over our own brave men. In spite of that, we took good care of these suffering soldiers.

These wounded soldiers were, as a rule, polite enough to us, and did not talk much with us about the actual war conditions. The reason of this was, as I learned later, that they really did not know much about them. Yet it sometimes happened that one of the younger German lads, or, it might be, some uneducated German farmer, forgetting that his life was in our hands, out of overweening Teuton pride, would endeavour to show us weak, defenceless nurses his strong love for the *Kaiser*, by sketching a rough portrait of him on the wall of his room, with the word "Paris" near it; and then the likeness of Napoleon, with the word "Waterloo" underneath. These were moments hard for us to bear, and though by our forced calmness, we showed no outward indignation, yet, inwardly, we were not lacking in resentment.

In the beginning of September, 1914, the German Red Cross Nurses arrived, and they immediately replaced us in this Hospital Base. Our doctors and our nurses were dismissed, of course, and I went back to our *clinique* in the *rue de la Culture*, where I remained to help *Madame*. There was only one patient left, a Mme. De Vos, one of our laundry women, who had to undergo some operation. With the exception of hers, all the rooms were without occupants. Yet *Madame* enjoined us to keep the beds still prepared, as it was customary, and to have the rooms cleaned every day. We did not quite understand her reason for all this work, in a tenantless *clinique*, nevertheless we did as she bade us.

The personnel in the *clinique* at that time consisted of six pupil-nurses, together with the supervisor. Sister Wilkins, and myself. Besides Pauline and José, there were the housemaids, the linen-room and laundry help. Our other nurses were doing work in the different hospitals which Madame had started, and the school-nurses were still occupied in the public-schools of Brussels. We were all in excellent health, and only suffered from the quality of the food, which was beginning to be poor. In spite of all we had gone through, we were not very anxious; and even when Madame Marie DePage came to us from the Queen's Palace, she did not bring any unusually bad news. She, too, like ourselves, and Miss Cavell, thought that the war would soon be over. Such was the life we were leading in September, 1914, only a very few days before our most strenuous work commenced.

Notwithstanding all we had experienced, we had up till now remained like light-hearted thoughtless children, and though we could begin to see anxiety and sorrow in *Madame's* kindly face, still, we did not yet fully realize the gravity of our situation; nor did we foresee the terrible fate that was impending over the principal personages of our humble little *clinique*. We did not even give the least thought to what might happen to us all. But, that evening, when we got hold of an English newspaper, in which it was made clear to us that at Charleroi, in Belgium, the English and the French soldiers had been obliged by overwhelming numbers, to retreat into France, our long cherished dream of a speedy conclusion of the war faded rapidly away, and we were again plunged into a state of despair. *Madame* no longer essayed to cheer us at her piano with her music and her songs, but, instead, she would talk to us every night about our duty to help the wounded soldiers, a duty that we could, at that time, with difficulty understand, since there were, as yet, no injured or maimed troops, in the *clinique* for us to nurse.

It was on the 26th of September, 1914, that *Madame* called us to her office, to explain to us that the German army had reached the French frontier, and also to inform us that many Belgian soldiers were at that moment without food and shelter. She, moreover, told us that it would be a very worthy and charitable act for us to give up our salaries to these destitute and hungry men. At first, we were quite surprised at this request; we had some difficulty in grasping her intention in wishing us to tender them our aid, for, until then, she had not shown any interest whatever in the matter relating to this horrid war. We were somewhat reluctant to part with the few five- and ten-*franc* pieces—the meagre amount of wages that we received from her—that we had to be very economical withal. Seeing our hesitancy she tried to persuade us, by stating that it would be a good way for us to show our self-sacrificing love and devotion to our unhappy country, in thus coming to the aid of these needy souls. She, moreover, added that she would herself take charge of the fund and relieve us of all the extra worry or responsibility that the good work would entail.

CHAPTER 3

# The First Refugee

We were now actually forced to realize to what an extent the war had reached, and how hard it was to bear the many evils that it brought into our former peaceful mode of life. We had, after the first excitement of the invasion, been getting used to war conditions, and as the seat of the actual fighting receded farther and farther from us in Brussels, we, like all the other citizens there, gave little thought to it, alas! Now, the frightful effects of real war were beginning to be keenly felt by us!

On the evening of the 27th,—a day that I shall always have impressed upon my mind—the weather was splendid, and the only thing that marred it was the continual distant booming of the cannon all around us. We were all seated at our supper, about 7 o'clock, with, as was customary, *Madame* at the head of the table. It had been a standing order of hers, that while at her meals, *Madame* was on no account whatever to be disturbed by any one. But that evening, however, her strict rule was destined to be broken. She was suddenly interrupted by Marie, her maid, who boldly entered the room, and in a low tone said something to her mistress that I could not understand. *Madame* arose, and immediately left the table.

Such an occurrence had never before taken place. We continued our repast, nevertheless; but as soon as it was over, we all proceeded to the class room, as was usual with us, and engaged in useful occupation. I was occupied with some needle-work, when *Madame* hastily entered the room, spoke a few words in an undertone to Sister Wilkins, then, turning toward me, requested me to follow her to her private room. I arose and accompanied her there. I can distinctly remember how many times I have gone to this identical room, whenever there was any momentous occasion for so doing, and how many moments I have spent there. As I was following *Madame* to her room, that evening, I could not help wondering why she looked so deathly pale and seemed so sad.

I little thought that, in a few minutes, I, too, would be looking just as pale and worried; and not without good cause; for before me, there were two nearly unclad, haggard, starving men seated in *Madame'* s office. One of the men appeared to me, at first sight, to be a soldier; but I could not then distinguish whether he was a friend or a foe. I inquired of *Madame* what she wished me to do. She merely said, "Take the young man who cannot talk, and whose name is Pierre, to room No. 9, and the other young man, who is called Louis, must be conducted to room No. 12, where he is to be taken care of by Mademoiselle Paula Van Bock Staele."

Obedient to her orders, I led, or rather, I half carried this ragged haggard-eyed, feeble, poor fellow to his allotted room, and gave him some food which he eagerly swallowed, as he looked at me with feverish blood-shot eyes. When he had finished eating, I laid him on a couch, and got a warm bath ready for him. His body was in a frightful condition from the hardships he had gone through, and there was also a wound that needed careful attention. He did not speak a word; but upon removing the remnant of what served him as clothing, I found an object, that was eloquent enough. There was an English flag wound round his breast! I instantly knew that he was an English soldier. That very moment I began to be anxious for his safety, and I thought then, as *Madame* told me later she also thought, that he must be concealed from his foes.

I knew not a word of English. All I could say was, "*Vous English?*"

"Yes, yes," he replied.

I was so upset about it all, that I actually forgot what to do. He looked up helplessly into my face, poor fellow, with such an appealing expression that the mere sight of it caused the tears to pour down my cheeks. He bent his head forward and kissed me on my hands.

"Whence did he come?" "Who was he?" I could not find out, not having a knowledge of English, which was evidently his mother tongue. He was a soldier, too, and would not speak a word, being bound by honour not to betray his friends. The other dilapidated and haggard looking man, his comrade in distress, was also an English soldier.

Needless to say, that this event threw us all into consternation, and this it was that had caused *Madame's* face to become so anxious and pale. In fact, it was a very serious matter—two English soldiers, allies of the Belgians, in our midst, and the city in the hands of the ruthless German invaders! Without our consent, and by force of circumstances, we were breaking the enemies' rules! Already, the latter, in red and black letters, had placarded on the walls of Brussels the following notice:

> Any male or female who hides an English or a French soldier in his house or on his premises, shall be severely punished.

Before this event took place, we used to read this notice without much concern, not fully realizing the gravity of its meaning; but, now, its full meaning burst only too clearly upon our minds. Here we were with two wounded and starving English soldiers in our home! What were we to do? We were hospital nurses, and surely, it was our duty to help these sick and wounded men; and help we must. But it was a serious case for us to undertake; and if I felt anxious about it, *Madame* also, must have certainly felt much more so than I. But, in spite of her anxiety, she decided to follow the dictates of humanity and fulfil her duty by taking proper care of these two unfortunate men.

Such was the state of our minds when we retired for the night, after having wished our new patients a goodnight. When I reached my room, I felt so tired that I immediately fell asleep, and did not even worry about the danger that lurked in our home. Our confidence in *Madame* was so great that we thought that everything she did was always right.

After having rested for two days, these two English soldiers both looked so refreshed and good humoured that it made us feel quite happy to see them. They were two as good-looking young men as one could wish to behold, and most of our girls were infatuated with them. We certainly gave them a very pleasant time, during the eight days they remained with us. We supplied them with cigarettes, and with plenty of English books. We had a most amusing time trying to converse with them; but with our limited stock of English words, we were greatly handicapped; we could only talk about the weather or the state of our health. Still we kept up a continuous fire of rapid conversation, after the French fashion, with the piano going most of the time, and managed to keep them gay and lively all the while. It was a pleasure to see their blue eyes brighten, and their faces break into a happy smile, as soon as they caught a glimpse of a nurse's white cap at the threshold of their rooms.

*Madame* came three times every day to their sick chamber to inquire after their health, and also to see if we were doing things rightly; and even Pauline, whenever she got the opportunity, would come and chat with the English patients, while Jack, the faithful shepherd dog, would mount guard at the door.

Meanwhile, outside, in the street, German soldiers would sometimes walk by, and cast a casual glance at our modest *clinique*, but without ever paying any marked attention to it, as there was nothing of a suspicious nature in the looks of the open windows and the wide open door of our home. These men were probably some of the advanced guard of straggling soldiers, who were on leave, and were enjoying a stroll through our suburb, after having enjoyed themselves with the amusements of the Belgian metropolis. But none of these men ever annoyed us, and moreover they were not very numerous; for at that moment, only a small army was left to guard the Capital; the great mass of the invading German forces was actually engaged in its rapid advance across Belgium into France.

So our English "Tommies" were not molested, and they remained with us for eight days, where, during the whole of that time they were royally entertained by us. One night, in the beginning of October, *Madame* told me to wake her at four o'clock in the morning, as well as the two soldiers, who were obliged to leave our place for some safer destination. She, moreover, ordered our Armenian boy José to prepare bread and coffee for the two men, and a lunch bag containing ten slices of bread for each one. I did as I was told to do, and, accordingly, the next morning at four o'clock, I found her ready dressed, wearing a blue cloak and a black hat. The two men were also ready and neatly clad in workingmen's clothes. After having drunk a cup of coffee and eaten a morsel of bread, they all went out into the still darkened street—first *Madame* and José, and then the two English soldiers, the latter following at a little distance. The two disguised Tommies seemed very brave about it, and walking boldly away, soon disappeared from our view.

We felt very sad at losing two such bright good fellows, who had brought so pleasant a change into our midst; and we were, moreover, sorry because we did not know what became of them.

Three hours later, *Madame* returned with José only. We understood by this that she had accompanied these men to another place of safety; and we were forbidden to make any further mention of the affair.

Immediately afterward *Madame* retired to her office, and in an hour or so, she sent for me to inform me that the next night we were to receive nine more men, and that I must get the beds ready for them. On the following morning, I happened to be opening the door, when a young woman of about thirty-two years of age walked into the sitting room and asked to see Miss Cavell; but, before I could deliver the message, *Madame* herself came to greet her, and led her into the private office, where they remained for quite a while. When the young lady came out of the office, *Madame* introduced her to me as being a Mademoiselle Martin, which was an assumed name, however, for her real one I afterward learned was "Louise Thuilliez." The lady then went away.

Later in the day, I saw Mlle. Martin again, together with the nine men who *Madame* had said were to be brought to our place. Of these nine men, eight were English soldiers, the remaining one was a Frenchman. How they ever managed to reach us without being noticed by the enemy, in the broad daylight, is more than I could, at that time, understand!

These English soldiers, of course, could not speak a word of French or of Flemish, and in these troublous times, it was rather a dangerous thing even for a Frenchman to speak his own language, with his accent so markedly different from that of the Belgians, without running the risk of being detected by the Germans. This risk was still greater for the English to run, as they could be more easily recognized.

All these men appeared to us to be very much worn out by the severe hardships which they had undergone. We hastened to minister to their wants. We prepared baths and gave them food, after which we helped them to their beds. All this gave us so much extra work that we were obliged to get the house-servants to help us in nursing these worn-out men.

That evening a young working man from the city called on *Madame*. She conversed with him in her office for a short while, then she presented him to me, saying, "This is Mr. Gilles, the guide." I looked at him, and, at first sight he appeared to me to be a man of about thirty-two years of age, rather poorly dressed, with a rosy face, and blue eyes that had a very honest look about them.

I could not understand where all these men had come from, and, as for themselves, they either could not or would not tell anything about their affairs.

I was brooding over this matter for a while, and after quite an interval of hard work attending to them, I summoned courage enough to ask *Madame* whether she would tell me whence they came. The look that came into her deep blue eyes, as she gazed into mine, will remain forever impressed upon my mind. After a slight pause, in which interval she seemed to be searching keenly into the very depths of my soul, perhaps with the intention of discovering whether I was trustworthy enough to be taken into her confidence, she decided to tell me the following facts: When the German army had advanced as far as Charleroi, a desperate encounter took place there from August the 21st to the 25th, and it is now famous in history as the "Battle of Mons-Charleroi." This we all know today, but at that time *Madame* only knew of the dogged retreat of the English and French, where, on account of the enemies' overwhelming numbers, and powerful artillery, many a brave young English soldier and many a French *poilu* lost his life.

It was about these agonizing days of terrible ruin and disaster that *Madame* spoke to me. After the gigantic human avalanche of German invaders had swept fiercely by with disconcerting rapidity, their commanders were too much engrossed by the vastness of their warlike enterprise to pay much attention to the casualties they had caused, during the preliminary battles they had fought in their quick advance toward the French capital. Thus it was that many an out-of-the-way battlefield where the British and the French had struggled with the enemy and lost, was now overlooked by the foe, as an unimportant detail, and consequently, many of these poor, wounded and worn-out soldiers of the Allies could be found scattered here and there over the numerous fields that formed the terrain of the recent early battles of the war. Some of these severely maimed and helpless men had managed to hide themselves away in some dug-out in the trenches, or in trees; others, more fortunate than the first, took shelter in abandoned farm houses, or empty stables; but many of them, alas! succeeded in get- ting to these places of refuge only to find there an agonizing and a lonely deathbed.

To add to the sense of utter abandonment of these ill-fated victims of war, the few peasants that had had the courage to remain on their farms, would not leave their shelters, to go to the aid of these suffering men. It often happened, however, that the children of the neighbourhood of these lonely battlefields would sally forth to reconnoitre, or to play, and be startled at finding a festering corpse of an unknown man lying in a ditch or under some brushwood where death had overtaken him. Whereupon, these frightened children would hasten home and inform their parents of their discovery. When night came, the latter would go out and bury these dead; and their graves would be afterward strewn with flowers by the hands of these same tender-hearted children who had been the first to find their occupants.

As I have said before, most of the farmers were afraid to go out to look for these men either living or dead, and I am sorry to state that, often, when they would hear someone knocking at their farm doors, late in the evening, the occupants of these homes would refuse to open. It thus happened that many a forlorn combatant deemed it useless for him to call upon the farmer for help; and even the children were sometimes afraid of receiving him because of the numerous detached troops that still remained in the small neighbouring villages, where these young ones saw every day some new proclamation against the harbouring of English or French troops thereabouts. We can infer from this how unhappy was the fate of these unfortunate men, whose rigorous lot was increased by the fear of the selfish farmers whose hearts had become steeled by the reiterated threats of their foes.

It is hard for Americans, who have been spared these horrors in their own home, to realize the saddening effects caused by the view of these humble graves upon the tender souls of the young children, who, sometimes, found as many as five or six of these dead bodies daily, in their wanderings over the fields; and you can consider yourself lucky, you who view those graves today, in the bright sun of peace, that you did not, like these men, who were flesh and blood like yourselves, die abandoned and unknown after many weary days of horrible anguish and suffering.

*Madame* went on to say that upon being informed of these sad cases, the Princess de Cröy and her brother, a bachelor, both of whom were at that time living in their *château*, on the French border, were greatly moved by the sorrowful plight of these war victims. These two charitable persons were very fond of outdoor sports. It was during one of their many trips across country that they either met with the children of that neighbourhood, who told them of the soldiers' plight, or they saw it for themselves. They immediately sent word to the Countess of Bellignies, a friend of theirs, who lived in the town of that name situated on the French border.

I have no knowledge of what passed between these persons, but the outcome of their meeting was, that they wrote to Mademoiselle Thuilliez to come to their home and decide what was best to be done to aid these men. As I have stated before, Mademoiselle Thuilliez was a

French teacher from Lille. I may add that she was a very brave and energetic woman, calm and self-possessed. She immediately determined to go to these places alone, to see what assistance could be rendered.

This lady personally told me how she went for the first time to one of these small villages, just above Charleroi. How she inquired of the farmers there, whether they knew of any refugee soldiers; but these men refused to talk to her about them. She then determined upon searching for them all alone. She waited for nightfall, then, accompanied by some of the children of the locality, she made her way to an abandoned battlefield. Here, there was no immediate danger to her person, because the Germans were then too much occupied and excited in their fighting elsewhere to give any close attention to these out-of-the-way places. The very ground they had struggled over was still wet with the blood of the wounded and dying, and encumbered also by all the debris of war. All this made it extremely difficult for a frail young woman like her, and for the tender young children with her, to tread their way in safety through the gruesome scenes of the combat of three weeks ago.

On Mademoiselle Thuilliez' first visit to these desolate fields, she failed to find any of the unfortunate soldiers; but on the second night that she courageously ventured there she saw a dark object lying half-buried in the slimy mud of one of the abandoned trenches. On closer examination it turned out to be that of an exhausted soldier in a dying condition.

Aided by the children. Mademoiselle Thuilliez managed to carry the suffering man to the humble cabin of some poor frightened miners.

After which she sent a messenger to the Princess de Cröy, who, the very next day, came in person to see the exhausted man. The latter was an English soldier. Upon seeing this charitable lady, he told her that many of his comrades were, like himself, lying wounded or dying in the trenches around about where she had found him.

After having found many of these disabled soldiers in the neglected battlefields of this locality, the Princess de Cröy, dreading to leave them in the villages, at the mercy of the selfish and indifferent farmers, had them removed to her own dwelling place; but she was unable to keep them there for any length of time, through fear of their being discovered by the Germans. She immediately sought aid from the Countess de Belleville, who was well acquainted with a Monsieur Capiau, a civil engineer of the City of Mons. The princess determined upon asking him, in the name of humanity, to help her take care of these suffering men, and to treat them as though they were patients. But through fear of their being recognized by the Germans, she also requested a certain Monsieur Libies of Mons, a lawyer, to furnish them with bogus cards of identity bearing assumed names of Belgian citizens.

Meanwhile, the Princess de Cröy, in the same manner as Miss Thuilliez, had discovered several groups of these wounded or exhausted soldiers at Wiheries, a small village in the neighbourhood of Mons. She, together with the Countess de Belleville, also asked a pharmacist of Paturage, by the name of George Derveau, to assist them in their undertaking.

After having come to a decision as to what was best to be done, they set to work, and succeeded in gathering together divers groups of refugee-soldiers whom by degrees they conducted to the home of Miss Cavell, in the *rue de la Culture*, at Ixelles, which place served as the central point of their reunion. These disabled and war-worn men were brought to our place through the following intermediaries: The men were first led by Miss Thuilliez to the Princess de Cröy's *château* in Bellignies, France; they were then taken to the house of a civil engineer named Capiau, by Monsieur Derveau, in whose house the fugitives obtained their bogus cards of identity. They were afterward conducted by various individuals of Mons, among whom were Madame Saduere-Tellier, Jeanne Dubuison, and others whose names have escaped my memory.

By reason of the great danger of their being discovered in the small dwellings of these persons, the Princess de Cröy, who was personally well acquainted with Miss Cavell, and had through the medium of Monsieur Bancq informed *Madame* of these undertakings, agreed with the latter to have the needy men brought to her place. This Mr. Bancq and a Mr. Severin had previously consented to receive these wounded fugitives in their own homes in Brussels, until Miss Cavell could find room for them in her *clinique*. There was also a Madame Ada Bodart, of Brussels, who had in the same way given refuge to some of these unfortunates, whom she, too, kept with her until Madame Cavell was ready to receive them.

These groups of tired and disabled soldiers soon began to arrive at our *clinique* in the *rue de la Culture*, all brought there by Mademoiselle Thuilliez. After they had received proper treatment from us and when they had sufficiently recovered from their wounds, or their fatigue, they were sent away to a place of safety in the direction of Holland. Upon leaving Miss Cavell's home, these men were placed in the charge of the Belgian guide, Gilles. This trusty man managed to conduct his charges as far as Antwerp, where another guide would relieve him of his responsibility and lead them to Turnhout, a village on the Dutch frontier, over which by means of certain men and women, to whom they were directed, and through the payment of the sum of one hundred *francs*, they were safely led into Holland. They found no difficulty in paying their way across the border, since they had been plentifully furnished with money for that purpose by the generosity of Miss Cavell herself, and of Mr. Severin, of Brussels, and many other brave and kind people.

Directly these fugitives got into Holland, they were at liberty. Once there, many of them found their way to England or to France, where those among them that were not disabled, might again take their places in their respective armies.

Such were the events that had happened during the first stages of the war, leading to the advent of the exhausted soldiers at our *clinique*,—all which occurrences *Madame* related to me in her usual calm and dignified manner, as she took me into her confidence. Everything she said contributed towards showing me how strong this astonishing organization for the saving of refugees' lives really was; though I, myself, at that time, could not fully comprehend it.

When *Madame* had told me all that she thought important for me to know, she further showed her trust in me by adding that she considered me as her friend and partner in this undertaking, and also cautioned me against speaking of it to the other nurses. She then left me, and I went to the small room to see to the nine men, all weak and exhausted, that had been placed under our care. These men, already mentioned above, seemed to be in a pitiable state, indeed, and they were far more depressed in mind than the two English soldiers whom we had first received. However, we had orders to do the best we could to cheer them and to make them feel as comfortable and as happy as we possibly could. All this gave us much extra work, but we all did our best to fulfil our duty in the cause of suffering humanity, and also to please *Madame*.

What I have to relate now may at first glance seem trivial, and gossipy, but it is necessary for me to state it, as it led to serious consequences. It is as follows:

When we had succeeded in restoring these poor men to health, and had dressed them in clean clothes, they appeared so much changed and attractive that they could not fail to impress one with their youthful, manly air. It happened that one of our nurses, a young and pretty Russian girl, by the name of Dora Betsis, who had helped in the nursing of two of these young English lads, suddenly seemed to grow very fond of them, and they in their turn, showed a great liking for her, to the extent of being jealous of each other. They both manifested their affection for her by writing verses and other trivial thoughts in her autograph album, and they even signed their real names to these inscriptions.

All this seemed innocent enough, to us all, and in all probability it was so intended by these young men; but it was a very dangerous thing to do, in these war times, and we eventually had to pay a terribly dear price for this most imprudent act. However, nothing immediately happened, for when they were well enough to go away from us, they, like those that had gone before, were, one cold, frosty morning, at four o'clock, led to another place of safety by *Madame*, and José, and her good dog, Jack.

The nights had been growing gradually colder during these several trips, and Miss Cavell appeared more thin and frail after each of them, and it seemed to me that for a woman of her age, these chilly morning trips did not benefit her health in any degree. But who can tell what was passing in her mind, and the extent of suffering this proud and charitable soul was undergoing in her sad and painful solitary struggles amidst these scenes and people that she had loved so well?

When, at six o'clock, she returned from her trip, she quietly took her place at the head of our breakfast table, where the meals were beginning to diminish in quantity as well as in quality. But, I am sorry to say, our young nurses didn't seem to realize the amount of fatigue *Madame* had to endure in these early morning tramps with the recuperated men; but one could notice the ill effects of them, by the increased depths of the lines about her mouth, when, with a clear searching gaze she glanced around at the assembled nurses to convince herself that they were all right.

From day to day, many more men came to our place, conducted there by Mademoiselle Thuilliez, most of the time, though some of them were brought there by Gilles, the trusty guide. We continued to care for these unfortunate soldiers in spite of the fact that more proclamations had, in the meantime, been made to the Belgian people, forbidding them to either help or harbour any French or English fugitive soldiers. We thought that it was our duty as hospital nurses to care for these patients, and we were also impelled to do so through our love for our mistress, whom we wished to help in her highly humanitarian and charitable work, without troubling her with any considerations of money matters.

At times, however, *Madame*, seeing our fatigue, would advise us to go for a walk in the fresh air, and she would sometimes send me with a letter to Mr. Severin's house, a trip which gave me a greatly needed change.

The reader must not imagine that all these comings and goings could go on unobserved by everybody. It was not long before the Committee of our *clinique* began to suspect that something unusual was occurring in the *rue de la Culture*. But as Madame DePage, one of its members, who was personally interested in Miss Cavell's enterprise, seemed to have a share in the wounded refugee-work, they did not dare to interfere with it, though, as I later learned, they highly disapproved of it all.

During all this period, the buildings of the New *Clinique* went on under construction, and *Madame* went still, from time to time, to view their progress. She had so longed for their completion, and for days and days she had spoken of them to us, telling us how much cleaner and brighter the new home would be and how much easier our tasks would be.

This was towards the end of December, 1914. By this time, our friends in the Metropolis were becoming more and more excited, and indignant against the tyrannical invaders. On every occasion the City of Brussels was forced to pay great sums of money on account of these manifestations of ill will on the part of its citizens against the foe. These fines only served to increase our hatred for our hard taskmasters.

# CHAPTER 4

# Christmas 1914

About Christmas time of this same year we had received several more men in our *clinique*. Among these was a certain English commanding officer. I had never seen such a handsome, noble looking face as his, among all those men who had come to our home. He soon became a great favourite with everybody, and was the ideal of the nurses, and he also seemed to have become the right hand of Miss Cavell, in directing the other men, and in organizing parties and entertainments for the Christmas holidays. He took much interest in these events, and personally assisted in their preparation. It was he who gave *Madame* the idea of asking some homeless children of the city schools to share our Christmas dinner. This she did, and when the festive day arrived we had as many as fifty children in our home, and all of them with hungry stomachs and big shining eyes, looking covetously at the many good things spread before them on our tables.

It was also this handsome, gallant officer who opened the dining room doors to these expectant young ones and conducted them each to their chairs, giving them all a hearty welcome. He then took his place at the head of the table, next to that of *Madame*. When the children and the rest of those who were present had done justice to our hostess' hospitality, this English officer, whose command of our language was not very great, made us a short speech with a very marked British accent. He told us how solemn and beautiful the occasion seemed to him, and his brother soldiers, united as they were under our friendly and hospitable roof; and how grateful they were to us. We could not refrain from a thrill of emotion when, with overflowing souls the Englishmen with one breath loudly exclaimed, "God bless you all!"

Everything went off splendidly, and the festivities ended by everybody joining in singing the British National Hymn of *God Save the King!*

At midnight the children returned to their homes, with their stomachs well filled, and with happy and grateful hearts. Thus was the ordinary routine and drudgery of our lives relieved by a few happy moments like these.

These pleasant moments would soon be saddened, however, by the sudden departure of our newly acquired guests. So it happened in the case of our good-hearted British officer, for, on the very next day, at four o'clock in the morning, he, like the others had done before him, left our hospitable '*clinique* under the guidance of Miss Cavell and José. I never heard of him since, nor did I ever even know his name, and though he had promised to write to us, his longed-for postcard, which was to tell us of his safe arrival in Holland, never reached us.

Life in Brussels was becoming more and more miserable, through the vexatious measures of the Germans, who showed us much hatred, and did everything they possibly could to make our Belgian people feel oppressed and unhappy.

During the Christmas and the New Year's holidays, too, when everyone usually tries to be happier than at another time, and when their hearts are filled with hope for the future, this ill-treatment seemed all the more difficult to bear. Some of these acts were preposterous! When we think that merely because a German invader had heard an innocent child sing a Belgian folk-song they tyrannically imposed a fine of 50,000 *francs* upon the city of Brussels. Added to this affront, from the first of January, 1915, it was forbidden for the citizens of that city to venture out of their homes after seven o'clock in the evening. Furthermore, all the gas mains and the electric lighting plants were cut off, so that the poor inhabitants were left without light other than that of candles; and to make matters still worse, the principal reservoirs of the Belgian metropolis had been emptied of their contents, thus leaving the people without good drinking water.

Everything seemed so sad, but in spite of it all, the staunch Belgian people were still highly optimistic, and continued to labour under the belief that their troubles and vexations would soon cease. Notwithstanding their predicament, however, the good people managed to find a secluded place in which to talk about their country's woes. I recollect, that when I went to visit my friends and my family, on the occasion of the New Year, I discovered them hidden in their cellars, under the light of a tallow candle, gathered around a table upon which were a few bottles of Belgian beer.

Here they continued to keep the flame of the old Flemish spirit brightly burning. These good-natured and kind-hearted people had remained unchanged through it all! Though they were very sad at their unhappy fate, they still looked forward to better times! Galled and oppressed as these people were, they had to dissimulate their resentment, but notwithstanding the fact that under their troubles they continued to show a happy child-like smile on their face and a kindly beam in their gentle blue eyes, the German Governor knew full well that he had no mere children to deal with in the Belgian people.

Of all the cities which have been severely punished by these Germans, I believe that Brussels was the one that suffered the most.

On the third of this same month, things were a little better, but we still remembered the unpleasant cold and dark days which we had gone through.

Quite a number of English soldiers, many of whom were unwounded, continued to come to our place, and we busied ourselves as ever, in caring for them and in mending their soiled clothes. We endeavoured in every way to cheer them and to set them on their feet again. Our *clinique* in the *rue de la Culture* remained all this time quiet and forgotten. The Germans up to this time had not suspected that our little home was lodging such great enemies. But this state of things could not last like that forever. It happened, at times, that some of our young men, feeling the need of fresh air, would imprudently venture outdoors, where passers-by could see them seated in arm chairs at the front door, enjoying the early morning air and the bright sunshine.

This was an innocent enough act, on their part, but it was fraught with much danger to us and to themselves, for in so doing they ran great risk of being recognized by the Germans, because those English soldiers could not dissimulate the hatred that showed in their eyes as they beheld any straggling enemies' soldiers, which could not fail to be noticed by the latter and arouse their suspicion. *Madame* was not slow to perceive the danger they incurred, and she decided to keep these men more confined, to screen them from the public gaze; and she would only permit them, in fine weather, to go for a short walk, accompanied by José.

Up to the end of January nothing of note had happened. Miss Thuilliez came at regular intervals, bringing men and news with her to our *clinique*, where things were going on all right. *Madame* had taken some extra help. She had hired a woman and two girls, to aid us in the kitchen and in the housework.

In the month of February several French soldiers came to us, and we treated them with as much care and attention as we had the others, and soon nursed them back to health, aided in this by the fine weather and the cold bracing air. It was not long before they began to show their Gallic temperament by becoming restless and venturesome. They took short walks in the neighbourhood, and as your French soldier, like his Belgian brother, is very fond of a glass or so of wine, it was not very long, either, before they spied a snug little *café* in the *rue de la Culture*, with the sign "*Chez Jules*" over the door. They did not fail to enter, you may be sure, and indulge in their favourite beverage. Very soon the English soldiers also got wind of it, and would often accompany the Frenchmen, promising to behave themselves and not betray their identity. *Madame* did not mistrust them, and permitted them to go.

But her suspicions and her fear were aroused when one of these Englishmen came home in an advanced state of intoxication. You can easily imagine how shocked *Madame* felt about it, and how imprudent and dangerous it must have seemed to her! Moreover, she was powerless to hinder it. She had the man confined to the house; but, I, myself, saw this particular soldier, whom we had carefully hidden away from the peering eyes of strangers and enemies, talking aloud and drinking wine in an ordinary cafe. Who could tell whether some silent agent of the enemy might not be seated in such a place? If such a man were there he could not fail to notice the difference between the vivacious exclamations of the French soldiers and the slow, drawling accent of his British companions, with their broad smiles; and contrast both of these with the Belgians around them. With these doings, it was not long, you may be sure, before the whole neighbourhood knew that Miss Cavell was harbouring French and English soldiers under her roof.

When the time came for these men to depart for Holland, we were glad because we were commencing to fear that they might bring trouble upon us; and it actually happened, one or two days afterward, while I was taking the air in one of the streets near our *clinique*, that I noticed two German officers who seemed to look at me very closely. This made me feel nervous, knowing as I did that our place was full of English soldiers.

I began to keenly realize the danger we were incurring in harbouring them. Notwithstanding, I endeavoured to assure myself that there was nothing to fear, that perhaps my imagination was getting the better of me.

An important event, causing much sorrow to us, happened in the month of March. From the beginning of hostilities to the present time, the Saint Gilles' Hospital had been occupied by our own Belgian sick, and during that interval these patients, as we have already said, had been treated by many of our own nurses. But, as was always the case with them, the German invaders requisitioned the Brussels hospitals for their own sick and wounded, and it was not long before all the Belgian patients were transferred to the St. Jean's Hospital in that city. It also followed that all our nurses were, on account of this, left without work, a thing which made them very unhappy. In hard times like these, too, it was very difficult, if not impossible, for them to obtain another situation. Upon hearing of their misfortune, *Madame* bade the nurses not to worry about it, and moreover, promised to help them. She allowed them to remain with us; this increased the number of our personnel in our already overcrowded house, and also had for effect the rapid diminution in our food allowance.

During the same month, Madame Marie DePage left Belgium for America, to seek help for the wounded soldiers at La Panne and at Verdun. She bid goodbye to *Madame* with tears streaming down her cheeks. Did she already feel that this was to be the last time that she would see both her unhappy country and her most intimate friend?

She left us all after saying farewell, and soon sailed on one of the Belgian Sea boats.

*Madame* sent ten of the nurses that had lately arrived, to France, with the intention of having them help in taking care of the many wounded on the Yser. She conducted these nurses in person to Antwerp, where, in an humble farmhouse, a room was in readiness for them. On the following day she went with them as far as the town of Turnhout. And here an incident occurred which set forth in a beautiful light the pious nature of this noble hearted and charitable woman. When about to take leave of her charges whom she loved so well, she reverently knelt down on the muddy earth of Flanders and gave them her parting blessing.

When, a day later, she returned to our humble *clinique* she seemed broken hearted. She also appeared to worry because she had not been able to find any food supplies to meet the wants of the lately increased number of inmates of her household.

We nurses who had remained faithfully with her now began to

feel the evil effects of these very hard times. We were greatly in need of money, too, and of many of the necessaries of daily life. We hardly dared, however, to tell *Madame* of this, because we well knew that she had enough troubles of her own, about which to worry without adding to them by relating ours.

I thought that I had hit upon a plan to gain money, I decided to give French lessons. With this intention, one day, when I had two hours' leave, I hastened to a book store to see if I could find anyone who would be desirous of learning the language. Upon reaching the place, and looking anxiously for notices with a list of names of such as might want lessons, what was my surprise to find that nobody in Brussels was rich enough to afford to take French lessons! I went back home feeling sad and disappointed. The thought had not occurred to me at that time, that the Germans would not have allowed any one to even speak French.

As we were young girls and were very much occupied with our English soldiers, we had little leisure to worry over such privations. We had recourse to the piano and to songs, both of which came in use to keep up the good humour of our guests. Much of our attention was also engrossed by applying ourselves to the learning of English from them.

The kitchen servants became interested in these men, and I may mention in passing, that the cook's daughter, a young girl who had not been very long with us, suddenly began a flirtation with one of them. I well remember when we warned *Madame* of it, how shocked and annoyed she was at such behaviour on the part of one of her servants.

In the month of May, we received quite a number of soldiers at a time, and among these there was one who informed us that he was of Polish origin. He became very ill while with us, and *Madame* was often at his bedside. For more than three weeks he remained with us and we often saw him occupied in writing.

After Miss Cavell had conducted him to Gilles, the guide and he went elsewhere, we found on the floor of his room a German letter in which this boy had written that *Madame's* house was a good one, but that he could not do anything that was required of him to do.

When we heard about this letter being found, the thought suddenly occurred to us that we had been harbouring a spy in our home! But through the kind treatment of *Madame* he had evidently changed his mind about betraying us.

I now felt certain enough that we were known to our German enemies. I told *Madame* about the letter, but she didn't seem to be much impressed about it for, as yet, she had not fully grasped its meaning.

A few days later she sent me, together with one of the nurses, for a day's leave. We both decided upon going to town to see the movies. Our supply of money was very limited, so we walked in hunger through the streets of Brussels, where the animation was great. Several marked changes had, however, taken place since my last visit. The one that struck me the most was the desolate condition in which the beautiful Palace of Justice appeared to us. This handsome building was boarded up all around and German flags were everywhere to be seen.

Another sight that caused the blood to freeze in our young veins, was that of the many notices with *Verboten* on them, pasted on the city walls; for we could not fail to see over a hundred of them, warning the citizens against harbouring an English or French soldier under pain of death.

Signs of oppression were to be seen everywhere, and many were the frightened faces that I met in the lower part of Brussels, where I learned that several persons, ignorant of having done wrong, had been recently punished, only for wearing a sprig of green holly on their dresses.

We went to the movies, where in a cheap place we viewed an American film. It was very interesting, indeed, and it made us forget for a while the unhappy conditions of the outside world. It was rather late, and far past the regulation hour when we reached home. The night-nurse opened the door, and bade us make no noise. "*Madame* is already abed," the nurse said, "and it would be best for us to go to our rooms without attracting her attention." We decided to go in our stocking feet, and taking off our shoes, we carried them in our hands, as with rapidly beating hearts we cautiously mounted the crooked stairs, for we were ashamed to be late, and sorry to displease *Madame*, who had placed much trust in us.

It was very dark on the stairs as we mounted, and when we were about half way up I felt something touch me against the wall. Before I realized what it could be, I heard *Madame's* voice saying, "Put on your shoes, my children; I'm afraid you will catch cold." In my fear and excitement, I let both my shoes drop on my feet, which hurt me much, but I did not dare to cry out. We went to our room feeling sheepish and tired.

Rue Darwin.

Street corner

VACANT LOT

garden

garden

Owners Garden

Cittrigure Edith Cavell

Madame's Office

Caffy

145  147  149  151  153  157  159  161  163

Picture Print Store

Garden

Café Chez Jules

Rue Berkendael.

Rue de la Culture

Potato Field in wartime
Before the war, used
To Drill Grounds By the

Belgian Soldiers

To the Depage Hospital

10 minute walk
20 minutes to the Chicaque

Yard or Gardens

Houses

The next day we were called quite early to *Madame's* office, where, after asking us to explain ourselves. Miss Cavell mildly admonished us, and warned us in future to be more prudent and to take care of our reputations. At first we did not attach much importance to these words, but, later on, we fully realized what they meant.

One evening in the month of June, shortly after supper, I went out for a walk in the streets immediately around our home. *Madame* was standing in the middle of a field before the *clinique*, where some poor people had for several days been busy planting potatoes. *Madame* went very often to look at them, and gave them some kind words of encouragement. Pauline was also standing by her, while Jack, the dog, was lazily lying on the grass.

While I was walking in the *rue de Berkendael*, a tall, handsome man asked me where the "Edith Cavell *Clinique*" was situated. The man's accent was of the most beautiful French that one could possibly hear, and his manners were those of a well-educated well-bred gentleman. He explained to me that he was a French soldier, and that he was looking for a hiding place for himself and a friend of his. I do not know what urged me to do so, but I gave him the wrong direction, and continued my walk; but while I was turning around a corner, I chanced to look backward. There was the French officer following me. Upon noticing that I was aware of his movements, he crossed to the other side of the street, where a man in a gray summer coat was standing. He spoke a few words to this individual, and then pointed with his finger to where Miss Cavell was standing in the very same street where the potato field was located. There was something ill-boding in this man's look and gesture, and, in my heart, I felt that all was not right.

Not knowing what else to do, I instantly ran toward *Madame*, feeling very nervous, and all in a tremble. I told her that a man whom she herself could see, was asking after her and the place where her *clinique* was. I added, that I was certain that he was a spy. She only laughed at this, and said that I always saw spies everywhere, and turning away she, together with Pauline, walked toward the entrance door.

In the meantime, the two men also approached the doorway, and I noticed that *Madame* let them enter the house. I was much worried at it all. Even Jack, the dog, raised up his head and appeared to be restless. We both approached the house together when the dog began to be very much upset. A few minutes later I was called to *Madame's* office, where she presented me to them both; the one as a Monsieur Gaston

Quin, and the other as a Mr. X, an Englishman. She asked me to look after Mr. Quin, and to put him in a room where there was a French soldier who had just arrived the night before, and had been comfortably installed. The other man, whom we called Mr. X, for lack of a better name, was placed in a room where several English soldiers were talking and smoking together.

Monsieur Quin was, as we have said, a typical Frenchman with perfect manners, and beautiful language. He was tall and very slender, his visage was adorned with what we call a Bourbon nose and his blue eyes were keen, yet soft and kindly in expression. It was not very long before all the nurses fell head-over-heels in love with him, but as they were very closely watched by *Madame*, they did not dare to show any outward signs of their infatuation.

The next day, the Frenchman told us that he did not feel well enough to leave for Holland. So *Madame* decided to keep him under our care for a week or two more. But early the next morning she conducted his friend and the others to Gilles, the guide, as was her wont. So that Monsieur Gaston Quin remained with us, and became the charge of all the women. Perceiving that he could obtain anything he desired of them, he requested them to accompany him for a walk when they were off duty. He seemed very friendly to little Pauline Randell; her broken French and pretty face made a strong impression upon him. He asked her also to go out walking with him; which she did, I believe, but it was only once.

Léonie, the cook's daughter, was in love with him, too, and even José, who had been married for some time, introduced Quin to his humble family. When José's first child was born about this time, its mother gave it the name of "Gaston," Monsieur Quin's first name. This gentleman became very friendly with the poor people who worked in the fields over the way, and it seemed to me that he had many conversations together with them that must have been of interest to himself. He seemed hail-fellow-well-met with everyone. But as I detested him from the very beginning, and was much prejudiced against him, I could not share in the general good will and liking that was shown to him. I attributed my dislike for him to be the effect of an excited imagination.

The guide Gilles came in a few days after and appeared to be extremely nervous. He asked to see *Madame*, at once, and while he was waiting for her, he was seen by Monsieur Quin, who eyed him in a very peculiar manner. Gilles informed *Madame* that Mr. X, the so-called Englishman, had suddenly disappeared from the group of men he had lately conducted to Antwerp, and he assured her that he suspected the man was a spy.

Gilles departed, but not before he warned us to keep a good watch on the street, and also upon everyone who came into our house.

That very evening we saw three strangers talking to the people in the opposite field. Léonie, the maid, was out with Mr. Quin for the whole afternoon, and a German officer, in his brilliant uniform, came to our *clinique* to ask for a vacant room for his son, who was very ill. All these incidents seemed rather suspicious to me, and the sudden entrance of the above mentioned officer caused Pauline and myself to tremble with fear, as it did all the other nurses. But after having talked with *Madame*, towards whom he behaved very politely, we noticed that He left the house without giving any signs of wishing to inspect the premises; moreover, he did not even speak to any of us.

The next day *Madame* again called me to her office, handed me a letter for Monsieur Bancq, but without any address upon the envelope, and bade me deliver it, remarking that it was very important. We had done the same thing several times before, without realizing what a dangerous thing it was to do. Even now, I thought nothing of it, and readily agreed to do it again.

While on my way to deliver it, I was walking along the *Chaussée de Waterloo*, where I met the ubiquitous Monsieur Quin. He had a cane in his hand, which he swiftly twirled around his fingers as he advanced. Approaching me, he asked me if he could have the pleasure of treating me to a glass of wine in a nearby *café*. This I politely refused, and gave him as an excuse that I had not the time to accept his invitation. I abruptly left him, and continued on my way without giving him any further thought. What was my surprise, when at the Porte de Schaerbeek, I saw him again, going in the direction of Monsieur Bancq's house. This time he did not look at me, but suddenly disappeared into one of the side streets, where there was a young girl awaiting him.

I began to feel uneasy, and was wondering if something evil was going to happen. A few blocks further on, as I happened to turn around, I noticed that a man had been following me since my last meeting with Mr. Quin. At first, I thought that this new individual was one of our Belgian boys, who had taken a fancy to me and, as is the Belgian custom, wished to accompany me on my way. Wishing to verify this, I stopped at a store window and pretended to be gazing at something inside. The man came up toward me, passed by without giving me a look, and also disappeared in one of the by-streets. When I had nearly reached Mr. Banrq's house, I again noticed this same individual talking with a German officer. I was afraid to go into Mr. Bancq's house, and, not to create suspicion, I decided instead to go to that of one of my friends. While on my way there I was followed all the time by this same fellow.

At my friend's home, everything was in a state of commotion. Just three hours before I came, the husband and the father had been arrested by the German police. It had become known to the latter that these two members of my friend's family had given shelter to some French soldiers.

Disappointed and anxious, I returned to our *clinique* in a melancholy mood. I did not even dare to mention any of these facts to *Madame*; I felt myself obliged to inform her that I had not delivered the letter to Mr. Bancq. Upon reaching the *clinique* I perceived Mr. Bancq himself, just as he was leaving our doorway. I was a little relieved at this, for I thought that possibly *Madame* would not ask me about the letter. I waited until the next day to return the letter, with the excuse that Mr. Bancq was not in and I did not dare to trust it with anyone else. I do not recollect whether she paid much attention to me, for at that moment she seemed greatly preoccupied.

The following day the weather was calm and beautiful. *Madame* went, as usual, to visit the New *Clinique*, which by this time was nearing completion. It was always a source of great pleasure to her to watch its daily progress. In the afternoon of the same day she went to the people across the way, and distributed apples among them and helped them along in their work as much as she was able.

Our house was, at this time, again filled with men, and Mr. Quin was still the same much-admired hero as ever. I had noticed him, several times, in the company of Léonie, who seemed to be very much in love with him. When, under the guidance of *Madame* and José, he finally left us for Holland, he seemed so sincerely sad at parting, that I actually felt sorry at having thought him so dishonest.

CHAPTER 5

# Suspected

On the tenth of June, *Madame* called us together, to inform us that in the following month we were to move into our New *Clinique*.

In the preparation for this event we were obliged to commence the furniture cleaning, and as *Madame* had no money to hire outside help, we had to do the work ourselves. This task gave the Englishmen, the Frenchmen and ourselves lots of sport working happily together.

It happened, one afternoon, that Pauline came in looking white as a sheet, and informed us, in a low voice, that two German soldiers were in Miss Cavell's office. We were quite upset at this, and we scarcely knew what to do about it. I decided to go to the parlour where I might perhaps find out something from hearing the conversation. Just as I reached the room, however, the two Germans left the house without even so much as looking around the place. Following them with my eyes, I saw them on the corner of the street talking to some of the people in the opposite field. I suddenly had a feeling that we were betrayed—that everywhere spying eyes were lurking, and that the men whom we had so carefully concealed were now menaced with serious danger.

At this juncture, *Madame* came out of her office, looking very pale. Instantly I ran up to her and asked her if all was well. With a wan expression upon her face, Miss Cavell told me that the two German soldiers had brought a letter from the German commander, in which it was stated that on May 7th, 1915, Madame DePage had gone down with the *Lusitania*. That was all it said, nor had Miss Cavell anything to say regarding my fears and suspicions.

At this moment Gilles, the guide, came in, and I imparted to him the news which I had regarding the two German soldiers' visit. He burst out into a forced laugh, and told me in his expressive Flemish language, that he thought we really were in danger—that *Madame* would tell us nothing about it, through fear of causing us any anxiety. Such was her greatness of character that throughout all those days of trial and care, she had kept her own sorrow and troubles to herself. It remained for the sudden fatal news of the tragic death of Madame DePage to tear away the mask of stoic indifference from that heroically determined face. It was with a sad voice and tearful eyes that she related the sad news to us.

We were all of us very unhappy about this sad event; for we had known the good-hearted lady very well. She had shown so much interest in our work, and now, without her to interest herself in us, we felt that we would be left all alone to incur the expenses of our undertaking, because all the other members of the committee were too much engrossed in their own affairs, or were, perhaps, too much annoyed by the Germans, to be of much help to us.

We began to be less gay, now, and we even did not dare to talk too loudly. We were also saddened by the war news, which reached us from time to time. We could hear the noise of exploding shells far away on the Yser River in Flanders. That was all the outside news we got, because nothing important was allowed to be published. But, we well knew that within a hundred feet from us, observant eyes were watching us, and quick ears were listening. We fully realized this; but, strange as it may seem, we dared not tell it to each other. To increase our plight, the food was becoming more and more scarce; meat and eggs were unobtainable, and we were reduced to the necessity of subsisting only upon bread and salads.

We went on, however, cleaning our furniture and preparing everything for moving day, constantly dreaming of our future New *Clinique*. This week, too, as was not very often the case, we were all alone, for there were no English or French soldiers with us to lend us a helping hand.

Mademoiselle Thuilliez had not yet returned, and Gilles was out with some other men that he was probably conducting to Antwerp. All that week, danger seemed to be lurking around every nook and corner of our dwelling; but, like thoughtless children, we too easily forgot our fears and sorrows.

On the twentieth of June, about ten o'clock in the morning, *Madame* received a visit from two men who spoke to her in English. They asked to see the house, stating that they wanted to rent the place after we had moved out. This sounded plausible enough to us, but I saw

# LA LIBRE BELGIQUE

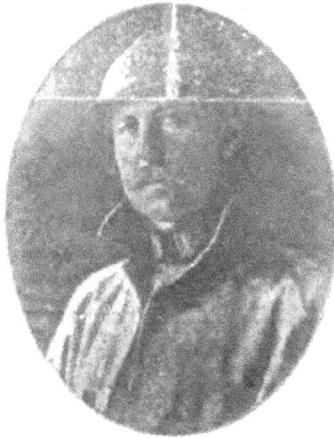

FIRST PAGE OF LAST ISSUES
OF THE FAMOUS FORBIDDEN PAPER

*Madame's* face become as pale as a sheet, as she allowed the strangers to enter. When they were mounting the stairs. Sister Wilkins noticed that one of the men wore army shoes, and had eyeglasses of German manufacture. She called little Mania Waschausky's, a young nurse, attention to it, and the latter recognized the fact. Both of the women became uneasy, when showing the men one of the rooms, where many English magazines and a few numbers of the *Libre Belgique* newspaper were carelessly left lying around. But the two men seemed not to notice all these details; and although they went through all the rooms, and looked casually at every corner of the house, yet they showed no desire of making a special inspection of the cupboards and wardrobes.

When we reached the bathrooms they examined the tanks. *Madame* was standing at the entrance of the room. Sister Wilkins and I were in one corner. Opposite the bathtub was a mirror and in that mirror I could plainly see the reflection of an English cap, which had carelessly been thrown into one corner of the room. At the sight of this object the blood seemed suddenly to stop in my veins—the room to swim round and round in my head. But no one noticed what I saw, and the two men soon left the room, engaged in deep conversation. Had they also noticed the cap? Who could tell?

After they had gone, *Madame* appeared restless, and for the first time I noticed how extremely thin she looked. I questioned her about these visitors, but she only said that they had been sent to her by her own landlord. That was all I could find out about them.

I did not dare to mention anything to her concerning the state of her health, or her sorrows. But remarking the extreme pallor of her cheeks, I ventured to ask her if I could help. She merely said, "You are a good girl. I am all right. Go back to your work, now, because, in a few days, we shall be able to move into our new home."

In spite of her calmness, we were all of us very much puzzled about the visit of these two men; but as we were busy about our house-moving and had plenty of work to think of, we soon for- got them.

On the 7th of July we received nine soldiers, all of whom were English. They had come in the night time and, as always, we gave them food and clothing. We warned them to keep quiet and not to go outdoors. So that, most of the time, they were assembled in one of our large rooms situated just behind *Madame's* office. This room was in house No. 149, and it had a door which led out to a small garden. It was also connected by a basement passageway, with houses No. 147, No. 145 and No. 143.

Owner's Garden

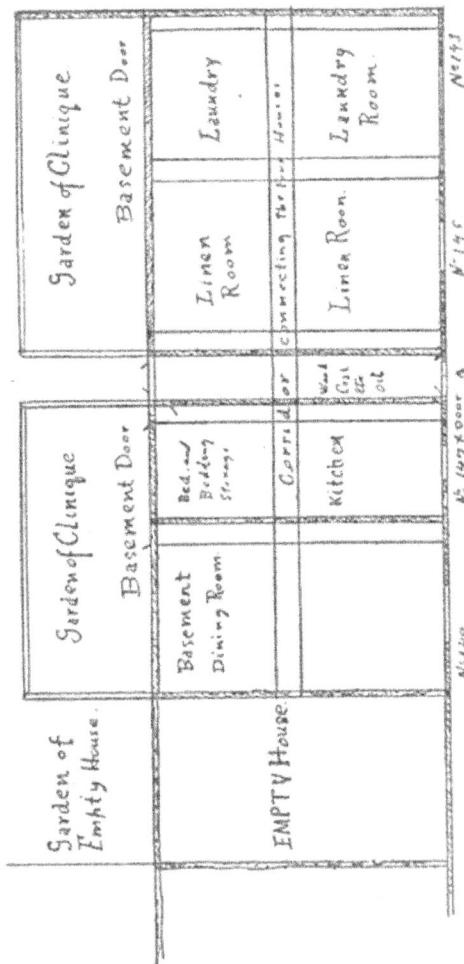

Garden of Clinique

Basement Door

Laundry

Linen Room

Corridor connecting the Houses

Ward Cut d d out

No 145

Garden of Clinique

Basement Door

Bed and Bedding Storage

Basement Dining Room

Kitchen

Linen Room

Laundry Room

No 147 Door

No 147

under the Proprietor's Entrance

Garden of Empty House

EMPTY House

No 149

Plan of Basement of the
Edith Cavell Clinique
Rue de la Culture

Ground-Plan of
Edith Cavell Clinique. Owner's Garden

VACANT LOT

Garden of Clinique.

Basement door.

Patients.

Patients

Patients' Hall or Sitting room.

Mad Wilkins' room.

Corridor

Corridor

Corridor

No 143

No 145

Proprietor's Entrance.

Leading into gardens

Garden of Clinique.

Basement door.

Class-Room.

Room where the English were Talking and Reading.

Waiting Room where the Books were hidden from all Night.

Edith Cavell's Office.

Corridor

Corridor

Wall

No 147 X Souri Portecachère

Matches went out again.

No 149.

Garden of Empty house.

Empty House.

Rue de la Culture. 1907—1915.

On the afternoon of the ninth of the same month, we were occupied in house No. 147, from which place it was not very easy to see what might be happening in No. 149. We were all talking together, at the time, but were suddenly disturbed in the middle of our conversation by the entrance of Pauline, who was making signs to us with her fingers at her lips, for us to be silent as, trembling with fear, she told us in a low tone that two Germans were in Miss Cavell's office, and that two others were outside the entrance door. In a second we saw the danger that the Englishmen were in, and we were ready to give our lives to help those men in that room behind the office in which the German police were making an inspection.

We were, in all, five girls with Sister Wilkins. Three of us went through the basement to the room where the men were in such great danger. The other two girls went out into the street, to talk with the two Germans outside. Only one girl remained in Number 145.

When we came to the room, the English soldiers were engaged in reading and talking. Sister Wilkins, who was with the three girls, put her finger to her lips to enjoin silence, and motioned for them to follow her without delay. The men saw by the expression of our faces that something unusual had happened, and, quicker than you can imagine it, they hastened after us into the basement. We opened the little door that led to the small garden, through which we helped the unfortunate men to make their escape. Once in the garden, they could easily jump over the stone wall and get into an empty house on the other side of it, that did not belong to us. The men were not slow to understand us, and before I could realize what was happening, they were gone.

For the moment, the danger was past, but who could tell what would happen next? What could the men do without José or Gilles for a guide? How could they get along without a knowledge of French in a country in the hands of the enemy ?

These thoughts flashed upon us like lightning, and Sister Wilkins went to José to ask him to roam about the streets to see if there was any possibility of doing something for the men in the vacant house.

Meanwhile, Miss Waschausky, Paula Van Bockstaele and I gathered together the different magazines, and were intending to put them under the bathtub. While we were carrying these precious objects in our arms, we were suddenly caught in the grasp of strong arms, and were told in a severe tone that we had forbidden objects in our possession. Trembling with fear, not so much for ourselves as for the nine men in the next house, we were at a loss what to do, so we burst into tears.

*Madame* was detained in her office by the two Germans, while the other two took us in charge—making us carry all the books and papers we had in our arms, they conducted us to the classroom, where they began to make an inspection of them. They had not been long making their examination of these periodicals which we had wished to conceal when they were interrupted by the entrance of one of the two men outside with a message in German. I began to realize that something had to be done by me, if I wished to discover something concerning these men. To effect this, I managed to get a step or two nearer them. You can imagine how great was my surprise upon noticing from my new position that the face of the man who had just entered was that of the very same fellow that had come to us the week before to wish to rent the place! I felt so angry and disgusted at this flagrant act of treason on his part that I actually felt as though I could have killed the man had I only been armed.

Not finding anything so very compromising in the papers we had, the Germans decided to leave us to ourselves.

At this juncture, poor Sister Wilkins, whose nerves had been so upset by what had so suddenly occurred, sank into a chair and burst out sobbing hysterically. The strain had been too much, and it had broken her naturally proud, calm, English spirit. We tried our best to comfort her, but all in vain, for her poor mind was in such a state that she did not understand our friendly intentions toward her. So we left her alone, and turned our attention to *Madame*. In this kind lady's office, everything was in disorder, the cruel intruders had rummaged every object that caught their gaze, and had strewn it along with others upon the floor. They had even taken Miss Cavell's family portraits from off the walls, torn them from their frames and thrown them, rent and crumpled, on the heap of ruins together with many other family souvenirs.

In the room in which the nine Englishmen had been an hour before, everything, too, had been wrenched from the walls, and the inspectors had been in such haste to discover the whereabouts of the fugitive soldiers that they had even smashed some of the windows. The Germans were now engaged in a thorough search of the entire *clinique*. Every nook and corner, every cupboard and closet, was carefully ransacked by them. When they had finished their inspection, they proceeded to question the maids so minutely and so often that they made the poor creatures very nervous and frightened. They burst into tears and were unfit to answer any questions.

During this interval, I managed to glide noiselessly to one of the attics to look into the street, with the hopes of seeing José. They had asked for José several times before, perhaps they guessed that he was helping in some of those acts that they qualified as forbidden. Glancing out of the window, I saw the other two Germans looking about them probably with the same intention. My heart beat loud and fast with excitement; but I was powerless to do anything! After watching the street for a short while, I caught a glimpse of José, but he was without the English soldiers. I inferred from this that he had seen the two inspectors, and had very prudently left the men he was with, for he immediately disappeared down a side street. The two Germans decided to follow the lad, and they, likewise, vanished around the corner.

Continuing to gaze at this same spot so full of interest to me, I noticed Pauline walking toward two men. Upon closely scrutinizing the latter, I was impressed with the idea that I had seen these two men before. To make matters sure, I descended to the front entrance of house No. 149. I arrived there just in time to see little Pauline talking to two of the English Tommies whom we had hidden that morning in our *clinique*, and who had just come into the street from the vacant house next door to us. Walking very slowly up to them in her simple childlike way, she disappeared with them from my view. I was somewhat anxious at this, for the direction which she had taken was sure to lead to the two German inspectors, and I feared lest they all three would be caught. The mere thought of this terrified me.

I re-entered the *clinique*. The two Germans inside were engaged in close conversation. After a few moments one of them went away. The remaining one began to make preparations to comfortably install himself in the front room of No. 147. He took a newspaper from his pocket and seemed, to all appearances, to be making himself at home.

In the meantime, we nurses had sufficiently recovered from our commotion to be able to prepare some food for *Madame* and ourselves.

Among the maids, I noticed Léonie, still trembling with fear and looking much paler than the others. She was most pitiable to behold. But I had no time then to pay much attention to her. I joined Sister Wilkins, who had sufficiently recovered, and we all went together to see *Madame*. We found her in her bedroom, also looking pale, but unchanged; she bade us see to everything, as usual, and to go and take our tea at five o'clock. When we saw her, calmly seated there, so small and frail, so peacefully quiet in her great trials, we almost felt as if we could fall down and worship her! But, alas! It seemed as though there was a gulf between us, so impressed were we by her stoic English nature; and we dared not remain with her in that bare miserable room. We felt so awed at her presence that we even dared not tell her what had become of our Englishmen. Perhaps Pauline or someone else had told her of them, or, maybe, at that moment, she did not fully realize with what great danger these men were menaced.

We returned to our dining room, and partook of a little food. We were glad when in a few minutes we saw *Madame* come down to us. She went to the kitchen and the laundry. She managed to tranquilize the minds of the servants and she also talked with us for a while, thanking us for having so faithfully helped her throughout these troublesome times. In a short time, order was re-established in our home in spite of the presence of that terrible German inspector in the front room of No. 147.

*Madame*, eventually, came to one of our rooms where she could better give directions to Miss Wilkins, as to what was best for us to do. "You must not show yourselves on the street," she said, "but must remain indoors as much as possible. The German inspectors," she added, "might possibly go away in the night time." Such was her conversation with us; it renewed our courage and stirred us to perform our various duties.

Shortly after six o'clock, little Pauline came back laughing and cheerful. Her happy mood seemed to be catching. I was nearly feeling quite like my old self again, when I, together with the other nurses, came to see her and to hear what she had to say. But so clever was the sly little English girl, that she did not betray her doings, nor even laugh at us for our idle curiosity. She merely turned her back upon us, and went on eating a thin slice of bread as though nothing had happened. That evening when I learned that José was back in his own home with his family, I went to the kitchen to find out what I could concerning Pauline. It turned out, as I was certain it would, that the latter had helped the two Englishmen to a place of safety in the house of an humble Belgian watchmaker, who lived in the *Rue de Miroir*, in Brussels. This man had accepted the poor fellows, and had concealed them in his own home.

How had this high natured little girl found out about this individual? Who told her that he was willing to help her? This was more than we could tell. It only went to show what a shrewd little woman she was!

She was also full of fun and playful mischief, and she did not lack it on this occasion. Here is an instance of it which she did not relate herself, but which we learned later. Every time she had to pass the room in which the solitary German was comfortably installed, an event that occurred at least some twenty times a day, she never said a word to him, but she also never failed to stick out her tongue at him. The burly Teuton would only look at her in return, with the air of a man that frowns at a naughty child.

When the evening of that wearisome and nerve-trying day at length came, we were all of us glad to retire to our bedrooms. We stood in great need of rest. In spite of the presence of that German inspector, who still continued to sit, all alone, in that front room, we were again beginning to feel more at ease.

Nevertheless, we decided among ourselves that it would be prudent to have Mania Waschausky, the night-nurse, keep watch over the front door of No. 149. She could easily do this, as I had done before, from the attic window; and if she happened to set eyes on some of our fugitive soldiers who might be returning home, she could try, by way of Number 143, to get them into the house unobserved.

So seventeen-year-old, little, black-eyed Mania, with her beautiful Russian face, made herself ready to keep a good lookout upon the different entrances of our *clinique. Madame* had also gone to her bedroom, and was perhaps at that moment offering up prayers for the safety of those hungry and homeless Englishmen who were wandering about the streets of Brussels.

The wind was from the west, and we could distinctly hear, from a hundred to a hundred and sixty kilometres away, the monotonous sounds of continuous cannonading, and even see the blood-red glare of the artillery fire that illumined the whole sky of the western frontier, where our brave fathers and brothers were nobly giving up their lives for those whom they had been forced to leave behind. What with the noise, and the day's excitement, my nerves were so irritated that I was unable to get a wink of sleep. I really think that none of us were able that night to do much sleeping, with the horrid fact tormenting their minds that a burly German was keeping watch in our midst.

I decided to go up with Paula Van Bockstaele and observe the enemy's quarters, so we glided noiselessly to the room in Number 147 and listened. What a sense of great relief we experienced when we heard the stillness of the place broken by the deep snoring of the German guard.

Paula, the sweet-faced little Belgian girl, went to the door of No. 143 to watch the German there, while Mania and I were both vigilantly leaning out of an attic window. This was rather hard work for us, and the awkward position nearly wrenched our bodies out of shape. But we dared not retire, for we instinctively felt that something would happen. It was now about midnight, and we had been for some time in this painfully uncomfortable posture, when we were repaid for our trouble by a glimpse of three shadowy forms making towards our *clinique*. We at once recognized them as being three of our men. The thought instantly struck us that they would betray their presence by ringing the door bell! How were we to prevent this from happening?

It did not take a second for Mania hastily to abandon her observation post, run as noiselessly as possible to the basement of No. 143, open the front door, and wave her handkerchief for the men to approach. When they drew near, she gravely pointed to their shoes, without uttering a single word. They took the hint, and quickly and noiselessly removed their foot-gear, and followed her into house No. 143. The poor fellows looked like emaciated ghosts, so terrible had been their sufferings since the afternoon they left us. Paula Van Bockstaele and I were trying to conceal the men as noiselessly as possible, in a large wardrobe in which we used to keep operating-room linen. Mania had, in the interval, disappeared and was now watching the German in No. 147. I went to *Madame's* room, to notify her about what had occurred and to ask what was to be done with the poor Tommies. Paula was busying herself in the kitchen, like the good girl she was, preparing food for them.

When I reached her room, *Madame* was kneeling before her bed, engaged in prayer. Upon seeing me, she quickly arose, and listened to my story. Suddenly interrupting me before I had time to finish it, she requested me to help her get out of the house to conduct the men to Monsieur Bancq. Dressed in her blue uniform, which consisted of a little blue coat, a blue dress and a hat of the same colour, she was soon ready to enter upon this new and perilous undertaking.

Silently I accompanied her on tip-toe through the basement, and let her out into the street, where, on the corner, she awaited the arrival of the men. Mania and I then led them to the door, where in eloquent dumb-show we pointed out *Madame's* dim figure in the darkness. The sight of her was enough for them, and they confidently followed her, just as so many others had done before, and they quickly vanished in the sombre night.

Now that we were certain that the men were safely out of the house, our thoughts reverted to the German on guard. We now became suddenly very much afraid of him, and none of us dared to go to that room. We wasted a whole hour before we could summon up courage to do so. Our little Mania was the first one to show her bravery, and she suddenly resolved to go there all alone. After a few minutes, she returned to tell us that the inspector was still there, but that he was, now, wide awake, and moreover he was very hungry.

I had not even seen the man, not daring to show myself, because I knew that he was aware of the fact that no one but Mania, the night nurse, had a right to be up and on duty. We could not tell whether he was asleep or not, during all these occurrences. Who could tell what he was up to or what his thoughts were? Perhaps, his only thought upon seeing Mania's pretty, smiling face, was of his own wife and children in his Fatherland!

At six o'clock in the morning *Madame* entered exhausted. She looked haggard and pale, while she told us that she had walked all the way, a distance of six miles, to and from Monsieur Bancq's house. She appeared so weak that it made Sister Wilkins cry to see her. We helped her to her room and put her to bed. We then gave her some coffee which seemed to restore her a little. She could scarcely speak. She could only make signs of yes and no with her head. She was cheerful, however, and oh! the happiness that shone in her eyes—and from her inmost soul! It plainly told us that she had again helped to save some unfortunate men from falling into the hands of their enemies, and felt fully repaid for all her trouble!

The German downstairs had seen Miss Cavell come in. Thank God that he did not ask us any questions. At seven o'clock he left the house. We were no further disturbed that day and we began to breathe freely once more.

But unfortunately this happy state was not to last long, for menacing clouds were lowering over us. The invisible but subtle web of surveillance was slowly but surely drawing its cruel meshes around our former peaceful home.

Such was the strain on our nerves at this period that the least thing was enough to frighten us. When *Madame* entered the room to tell us of her intention to visit the New *Clinique*, we all weepingly begged her to remain with us. We were afraid to be left alone. Even Jack, the dog, kept up a continual moaning, and Pauline, too, appeared frightened. We all of us felt downhearted; the maids and the cook sat pale and forlorn in a corner of the kitchen, and José himself was so sad at what was happening that he actually forgot to smoke his customary cigar.

It is impossible for me to describe how startled we became at the least little event. We nearly collapsed when the baker came in the morning. Whenever Pauline heard the door bell ring, she would become so nervous that she could scarcely move her lips to answer the caller. We were all of us in terrible dread of another descent of inspectors upon our dwelling. By this time, too, the whole neighbourhood had got wind of the German inspectors' visit, and it was all the talk at the Grocer's store. It seemed to us that the neighbours were all pointing their fingers at us, behind our backs. We were so timid at this thought that when we went to the new *clinique* to take, beforehand, some of the instruments necessary for the operating room, we ran like little children who are afraid to be alone in the road, as fast as our feet could carry us.

After a few days, however, we began to regain somewhat our former calmness. It seemed, again, as though we were being forgotten by the Germans, and we immediately began to make hopeful plans for the future. We set to work strenuously to clean and pack a thousand little things for our new home. José had already begun to paint the chairs and wardrobes. As *Madame's* means did not allow of her renting a moving van, we were all of us required to aid in the moving.

We began the work on July 12th, and each day we did as much of it as we were able to do. This was no easy task, I can assure you, for we had to carry many of the pieces of furniture by hand, or in a small hand cart.

On the fifteenth, *Madame*, in person, went with some of us to point out where our future sleeping rooms were located. She designated room No. 26 for me, and I shall never forget, upon receiving it, the impression made upon me by the fact that I had now to take care of it myself, learn how to make my own bed neatly, and keep the place tidy and free from dust. This in our old *clinique* had been done by the servants.

The moving of our furniture to the New Buildings progressed very slowly. It took us more than four weeks to accomplish it. Some of the nurses had previously entered into the new place and had made

Nurse Van Til
         3 slices of bread
                    E. Cavell.
12th of July, 1915.

it their sleeping quarters; while Sister Wilkins, *Madame*, I and some others, still remained in our old home.

On the 29th of July, Mr. Quin came back and asked to see *Madame*. We were every one of us in a tremble, for we thought it was dangerous for him to remain. We warned him that the house was under suspicion of the Germans. He assured us that he had no other place to go to. At sight of him, Léonie, the maid, nearly ran into his arms, while José's face fairly beamed with joy to see him. *Madame* also seemed very glad to see him again, and she promised to give him a room for that night.

The very next morning, Mr. Quin left us as suddenly as he had come, accompanied, as usual, by *Madame*, José and Jack. The separation appeared to me to be rather hard for him to bear, for he wept like a woman. We thought, by his actions, that he was afraid to go to the war, but I found out later why he melted into tears. It served as a veil for his eyes, to prevent him from seeing the noble woman who, drop by drop, was giving up her life's blood to pay for this man's love of ease and pleasure.

On the fourth of August, *Madame* received the visit of three men who said they were English; but she refused to receive them. She gave as an excuse that we were moving out. She gave them a card with Mr. Severin's address upon it. Alas! Poor Mr. Severin, the Brussels pharmacist! Poor Mr. Bancq! and poor *Madame!* Little did we think what was in store for them!

That same afternoon, we had another visit; this time, it was that of a German officer, who wished to talk to *Madame*. We nurses were much stirred up by this visit. We actually shivered so much with fright that we must have quite betrayed ourselves to him. We all lost our heads, and like little children, we burst out crying. Even Sister Wilkins could not remain quiet. Although Pauline told us that the man spoke very politely to *Madame*, yet we could no longer have confidence in any German. After a while the officer came out of her office, and took his leave with a polite salutation. Miss Cavell then came out seeming as calm as usual. We ran toward her, to learn something about the visit; but we could gather nothing from her sealed lips.

Some hours later, however, Sister Wilkins found *Madame* suffering from a terrible heart attack. It appeared that she had been subject to such attacks for quite a long time, but had always managed to keep it to herself. We did everything we could to help her, but unfortunately we were powerless to do much!

The next day she seemed a little better, and she informed us that the German officer had asked her if she had received any letters from the London war-office. He had looked over all her books, and found that the accounts had been neglected for three months back. He sardonically remarked that she must have had much to do to be thus prevented from keeping a good record of her money matters, showing thereby how crafty and knowing these Germans were, and how well aware they were of our doings; but cat-like, they enjoyed breaking their knowledge slowly to us, to worry us a bit, before finally pouncing down upon us. We became greatly alarmed when *Madame* told us that we must try to keep clear headed and cool, so as to help her as much as possible.

# Chapter 6

# Miss Cavell Arrested

On the 6th of August, we all of us were very much occupied with moving. We now had a little wagon with which to transport our furniture, and José and the maids were hard at work pulling the vehicle by main force to the new abode.

We nurses had also been very busy that afternoon, but were just engaged in talking matters over, when we were suddenly interrupted by the entrance of three men. They wore no uniforms, and we at first thought that they only wanted to examine some pieces of furniture which *Madame* desired to sell. But another glance at them was sufficient to show us that we were greatly mistaken. The expression on their faces was exultingly gleeful. They laughed and talked together in German, pointing the while at Sister Wilkins and Mania. I inferred from this that we were now fallen into the merciless hands of the Boches, who were gloating over the fact that we had finally been caught in their net.

They commanded us not to move, and pointing their revolvers at our heads, they roughly pushed us into a corner of the room. We now fully realized that we were prisoners.

At this juncture, we heard a low sobbing in the hallway; it was from little Pauline, who, seated upon the stairs in front of *Madame's* office, was weeping enough to break her little heart. Besides myself and Miss Wilkins, there were five nurses in all there. Their names were as follows: Sister Wilkins, Miss Waschausky, Miss Van Bockstaele, Helen Wegels, Fernande Weil. Sister Wilkins tried to escape, but one of the men led her to another room where she began to scream loudly and wanted to see *Madame*. We could give no aid, and were afraid to move from the spot. The suspense was terrible, the awful moments seemed to drag so slowly by.

Suddenly we heard the sound of several voices, the door burst open, and the figure of *Madame* issued, or rather was roughly pushed through the doorway into the room where we were, in the direction of the front door. Miss Cavell noticed us as she passed, and, pausing for an instant, made us see that she still had us in her heart. In spite of that hour of misery, she yet had time to think of what she could do to aid and encourage her nurses. In a calm and tender voice she said, "Don't be so sad, my children. Everything will be all right. I'll be back soon; be good and wise."

The German in charge of her put her into an automobile that was stationed before the door. The other men took Miss Wilkins and placed her in another automobile. All these events took place so rapidly that we scarcely realized what was happening. Poor Jack was howling disconsolately all the while, and some maids ran out of the house, but they were met by some other Germans who brought them back at the point of the revolver.

Things were in a terrible state now, in our *clinique*. We could still see in imagination *Madame's* calm face, so deep was its impression engraved upon our memories. We began to count the minutes for her return. "Would she come back soon?" we asked ourselves. We were all huddled together like prisoners and were not allowed to move from the spot. For five long hours we were thus detained, sobbing and moaning all the while.

It was four o'clock when *Madame* and Sister Wilkins were so suddenly taken away. At nine o'clock the latter returned alone. We were all of us eager to find out what had happened to *Madame*, but the poor sister was so terribly nervous that she fell to the floor in a fit of hysteria, screaming so loudly that some of the neighbours came over to look in at the windows to see what was the matter. Jack was continuously hovering around Miss Wilkins. Perhaps he realized what was being done to his beloved mistress.

One of the Germans at this instant announced to us that Miss Cavell was detained at the *Commandantur*. We were all very familiar with that name; it did not sound so terrible to us then, the *Commandantur*, or German Headquarters, and the edifice in which it was established belonged to the Belgian Administration, the members of which were at that time either in England or in France. These buildings were not very large, and were situated in the *Rue de la Loi*, opposite King Leopold's Park.

Prisoners were not kept for a long time in this place, as there was not room enough in it for them. After a fortnight's detention they were sent home, or to some other headquarters in Laeken. The treatment there was much better than in any other prison. Hence, when we heard that *Madame* was at the *Commandantur*, we felt somewhat reassured about her. When Miss Wilkins was able to talk to us, she told us that *Madame* seemed to be well treated by the officials there, and that, in all probability, she would be back with us the next morning or in the afternoon.

The Germans had, in the meantime, decided as to what they were going to do with us. They did not keep us shut up in our rooms, but allowed us to move freely about in our four houses. The only restriction we were under was that of having to ask permission whenever we wished to go outdoors. When this was granted we were invariably accompanied by a German functionary, who always kept close behind us. As one's existence constantly maintains its course even in sorrow, ours was no exception to the rule, and we were obliged to go about our every day work as regularly as ever. We generally performed most of our work in the morning, without any hindrance.

The next day our horrible nightmare recommenced, for we heard that Monsieur Bancq had been arrested at the same time as Miss Cavell, and that he had been sent to the St. Gilles Prison. We could not help thinking of his wife and children. How helpless they would now be without his protection in these troublesome times!

Yet we could not give much thought to them, because *Madame* was ever present in our minds, to such an extent that some of the nurses seemed still to hear the sound of her voice in the now vacant office. The morning slipped slowly by, and still we had no news of our dear matron.

That afternoon a new proclamation was posted on the city walls, stating that it had been forbidden for any one, man or woman, to aid or hide men of English or French Nationality in their homes under penalty of death. One of these hideous placards was placed immediately opposite our new *Clinique*. This was the first time we had seen it there, and how horrible seemed to us the purport of its words! Yet, even now we did not fully realize its fatal meaning, nor how closely it concerned us, as well as our dear mistress, the sound of whose footsteps we every moment imagined we could distinctly hear, and whose familiar form, attired in its blue uniform, we expectantly looked to see enter her office.

On the second day of *Madame's* imprisonment. Miss Wilkins re-

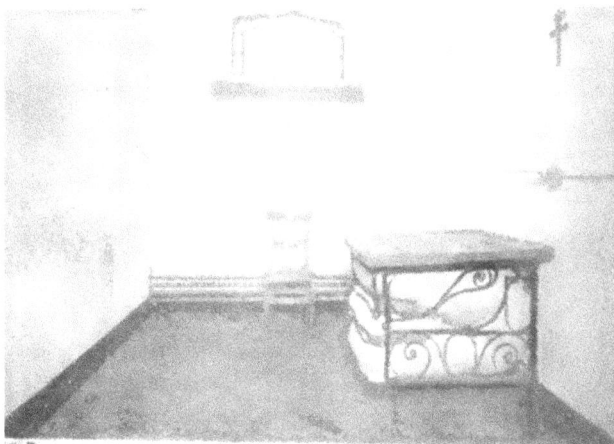

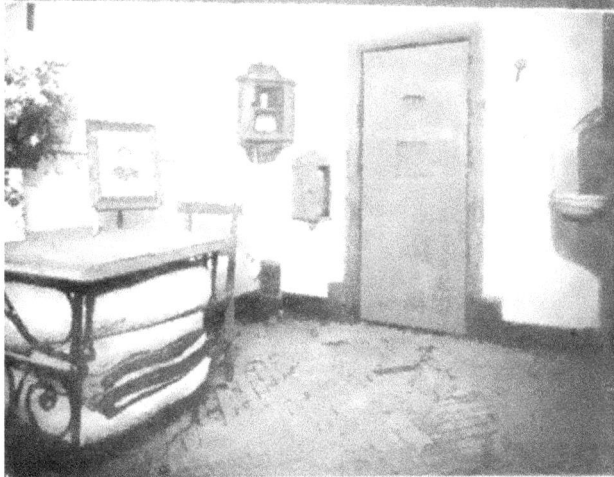

TWO VIEWS OF CELLAR
IN WHICH MISS CAVELL WAS IMPRISONED

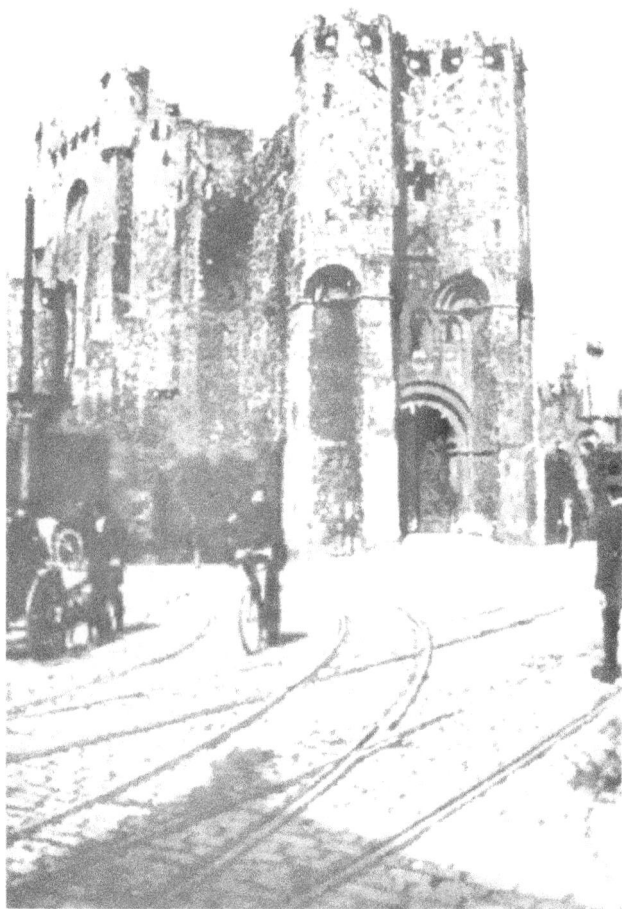

PRISON SHOWING DOOR BY WHICH
MISS CAVELL LEFT ON THE WAY TO EXECUTION

ceived a post card from the German *Commandantur* asking for some clothes and linen for our mistress. Sister Wilkins prepared everything that was necessary, and delivered it herself at the *Commandantur*. She remained away for some time, and when she returned she seemed broken hearted. She had not been allowed, she told us, even to see *Madame*, and moreover the German officers had treated her very rudely.

Several of us went there to see her also; but we all came back feeling very much disappointed. We, too, were not merely forbidden to see our dear mistress, but the German soldiers actually laughed at us when we mentioned her name.

On the following day we learned that the Princess de Cröy, the Countess de Belleville, Mademoiselle Thuilliez and several other members of that organization had all been made prisoners. We began to feel more and more anxious about ourselves, and being without a directing mind to help us, we became mere shadows of our former selves. We waited in vain for four days, but nothing came to enlighten us as to the fate of our dear mistress, and we felt as though we were engulfed in darkness.

Our housekeeping was beginning to be greatly neglected, many pieces of our furniture were stolen. The maids went out whenever they could, and Sister Wilkins was too sick to be able properly to take charge of sending out the furniture. José seemed very unhappy, and faithful old Jack would be lying the whole day long in front of his absent mistress's door.

The Germans were constantly in and around our new *clinique*, and when the day finally came for us to permanently enter the building, they deliberately accompanied us there, so suspicious were they of our movements.

Those were terrible days for us; God alone knows how terrible! It seemed to us, utterly in the darkness as we were, that everything was going wrong, while we were all alone without the good hand of our thoughtful mistress to come to our aid!

On the 10th of August we learned from one of the members of the *clinique* that Miss Cavell had been on the 8th of the month transferred to the St. Gilles Prison in Brussels. We could scarcely believe it. The mere word "Prison" was in itself so terrible to us; and it made us feel that something horrible had occurred to her. We wrote her several times, little nurses' notes, full of tenderness,—of innocent words, the outpourings of humble hearts. We counted our money; it was little enough, a few silver coins, and one or two copper *sous*. We bought

Yard.
Bakery
*Boulangerie.*

Hospital ward
*Infirmerie.*

Yard.
*Préaux.*

*Préaux. Yard.*

*Aile 5e Wing.*

*Aile 1re Wing.*

*Aile 4e Wing.*

Centre.
Middle.

E

W

N

*Aile 2e Wing.*

*Aile 3e Wing.*

Yard.
*Préaux.*

Yard *Préaux.*

*Cellule de Madame*
Edith Cavell's Cell N° 23.

Disciplinary cells.

*Greffe* Register's office.

*Blanchisserie.*
Laundry.

La Chambre où Madame
a été jugée *puis la dernière fois*
Last Trial Chamber of
Edith Cavell.

*Bureaux officiel.*

Jardin
garden.

*Cuisine* Kitchen.

*Cuisine*
Court-yard.

*Cuisine*
Court-yard.

Cour
Court-yard
*Guichet.*

Cour
Court-yard
*Donjon.*

*Jardin.*

Jardin.
Garden.

*Jardin.*

*Plan du rez de chaussée.*
Ground-Plan of St. Gille's Prison.

flowers with it; some roses and a bunch of white chrysanthemums—her favourite flowers! How carefully we selected them! Each nurse reverently touched each rose that was to be given to her. We sent them to our mistress, but, alas! we got no answer. We waited and waited for many days, but never a word did we get.

We knew from Dr. LeBoeuf, who had brought some patients to the new *clinique*, that Mr. Sadie Kirschen, a Belgian lawyer, was allowed to see her in her cell, and to take charge of her case.

In these sad and weary days, when a new housekeeper had been accepted by the committee to look after us, we had only one friend in whom we could confide or from whom we could ask information. This person was a lawyer, too, by profession, and a member of the committee. His name was Mr. Van Alteren. He did everything he could to help us, but he was powerless to do much because he himself was held in suspicion by the Germans, and when we stood most in need of his aid, he also was taken away from us and sent to Prison.

We waited during the entire month of August for news of Miss Cavell. None came. We began to feel weary. All interest in the *clinique* seemed to have died away. Everything appeared abandoned and different from what it used to be. For instance, all the servants, together with Pauline, had been discharged. The new housekeeper showed herself to be very strict. When we dared to ask her why Pauline was sent away, we were told that they only desired well educated attendants.

How dark and hopeless those dreary days appeared to us! With the cannon everlastingly booming in the distance and the pangs of hunger gradually but surely making themselves more difficult to bear, our sorrow and anxiety were all the more intensified by thoughts of our unfortunate Mistress in her prison cell.

We roamed around her prison whenever we could do so, to try to get news of her; but the Head Warden, a Mr. Marin, a Belgian, though he was an amiable and willing man, could do nothing to help us. We could only learn from his wife that the room occupied by Madame was No. 23. Nothing further could we find out.

September came, and still no news. Several nurses resigned, and new girls who had been accepted some months before by Edith Cavell, took their places; only a few of the nurses who had helped *Madame* in the Old *Clinique* now remained. Many changes had taken place in the New One, where the different papers were examined daily by several ladies of the committee, whom we scarcely knew. All these individuals seemed so different to us, and yet they were, for the most part, composed of the same members who were at the little *clinique* in the *rue de la Culture* when we received the fugitive soldiers.

About September the 14th, Sister Wilkins, at last, got a letter from Miss Cavell. How can I describe the eagerness with which we all crowded around to listen to the reading of the precious epistle! How its every word seemed to soothe and caress our ears!

It ran as follows:

Prison of St. Gilles,
Brussels.
14th September, 1915.

My dear Nurses:-

Your charming letter has given me much pleasure, and your beautiful flowers brought life and gay colours into my cell; the roses are still very fresh, but the chrysanthemums did not like prison life; they are like me; they cannot resist a very long time.

I am very happy to hear that you are attending to your work and that you are devoted to your patients and that the patients are satisfied.

I hope you will continue with your studies, just as though I were there, because in a very short time you will have to undergo an examination and I would like to have you ready for it.

The new term begins very soon; try to profit by your past experiences, always be prompt, because the doctors do not like to wait for their pupils.

Everywhere in life we learn something new and if you were in my place you would soon realize how precious is liberty and how grateful we should be to have it.

We must all learn patience. It is not enough to be a good nurse only, but you should also be Christian women.

It seems that the new *clinique* is very nicely arranged. I hope I will see it soon and all my nurses as well.

Goodbye, be wise and good.

Truly yours,
Edith Cavell.

This letter gave us a little hope and for the first time in all these sad days of our *directrice's* absence we summoned up the courage to play on the piano our national hymn, the *Brabançonne*, and the English one of *God Save the King*. But on the following day our ill-founded hopes

126

again vanished. One of the members of the committee, Mr. Heeger, a professor of the University of Brussels, who very often frequented the *clinique*, came in and expressed his opinion that Miss Cavell would be sent to Germany. Most of the members of the committee thought as he did. We could not believe this to be possible; but were still full of hope; and at frequent intervals, during the long days of anxious waiting, we could be seen gathered together, talking about *Madame*, and persuading one another that she would soon be back with us.

On the 21st of September, Mr. Heeger informed us that he had received another letter from Miss Cavell in which she seemed to be quite well and in high spirits.

Letter from Miss Edith Cavell to Monsieur Heeger:—

Saint Gilles Prison, Sept. 22, 1915.

Monsieur Heger,

Miss Wilkins told me that you asked me to write to you; it is with pleasure that I respond to your request; unfortunately I have not yet been able to send any letters.

I regretted deeply to have been forced to leave the school[1] at the time of our moving and to have left all my affairs in disorder.

I hope that now everything is well arranged and organized according to your desires.

I shall be very happy to see you a little later on; there will be certain things to be arranged, and I should like to have the opportunity to speak with you . . .

Please give my regards to all the members of the Committee, etc. . . .

Edith Cavell.

These little bits of information contributed to strengthen our belief that our dear *Directrice*, after a few months of detention, would certainly be released, as, from the perusal of the above letter we can infer that she herself thought she would be.

On the 22nd of the same month, we heard, through Mr. Van Al-

1. Miss Cavell alluded here to the transfer of the school for nurses in the little *clinique* to the new buildings which it now occupies.
École Edith Cavell
*École Belge d'Infirmières diplomées*
1914-1919
From
(Committee of Administration Report)

teren, that Maître Sadie Kirschen was no longer allowed to see her in prison. The German court had allotted her a new lawyer of their own nationality. This news made us feel very sad; it looked terribly ominous to us. Nevertheless, we, and even the members of the committee, had still some hope left of her return. The latter had done all they could to endeavour to communicate with *Madame*; but all in vain! The German hearts remained as mercilessly closed to pity as did the huge prison doors that cruelly enclosed our dear suffering *Directrice*.

# CHAPTER 7

# The Execution

About seven o'clock on the eleventh of October, while we were all sitting together in the schoolroom with most of our day's work done, we were talking as usual about *Madame*, and were still deluding ourselves with the hope of her speedy return. Just then, one of the nurses happened to look out of the window and recognized Mr. Van Alteren, who seemed to be plunged in a state of profound despondency. The nurse asked me if I knew why he appeared so worried. I could give no answer, however, but, impelled by I know not what, I arose and immediately ran to the front door, where the good gentleman was standing, with his broad shoulders bathed in a sea of golden sunshine that was striving against fate to make the grief-stricken *clinique* appear like a happy dreamland. There was something fatally tragic in the expression of Mr. Van Alteren's eyes, as I asked him, with a quick and nervous voice, if he knew anything about *Madame!* He did not speak a word; but entered with me the small library that was near the entrance.

Still, I could not realize that matters were any worse; but, when, in a voice choking with sorrow, he said to me, "Poor child! poor nurses!" I felt that the worst had come and that *Madame* was lost to us forever!

With a voice dry with sorrow and emotion, I intuitively gasped, "When?"

"Tomorrow at five o'clock," he answered.

I do not recollect in what state of mind I returned to impart the news to the other nurses, but, alas! they were already informed of it. Dr. Heeger, who had that instant heard the horrible news from Maitre Sadie Kirschen, had immediately told it to Sister Wilkins, who was wild with emotion at it, to such an extent that it was impossible for us to keep her in the house; she could not be tranquilized, but excitedly exclaimed that she wanted to go and save Miss Cavell.

We felt too miserable to pay much attention to her then, for, in fact, we did not know how to act. We had to try hard to keep cool ourselves under this great affliction. Oh! but they were sad and soul-wracking times! The memory of those agonizing days shall forever cling to the depths of my heart and soul!

Towards eight o'clock, however, we began to notice the absence of Sister Wilkins. She, being English and in a very excited state of mind, we were in fear that something serious had happened to her. We waited an hour for her, during which interval we thought over what we could do to save *Madame*. At nine o'clock Miss Van Bockstaele. Miss Buck, an English girl, Miss Waschausky and I went to the Prison. We had been there many times before and the kind-hearted Belgian, Mr. Marin, Superintendent of the Prison, had done as much as he was able to do for us. This time, too, he promised to bid goodbye to *Madame* for us, if it could be done, but he could not vouch for it, as there were two German Wardens on duty before her cell.

Upon asking Mr. Marin about Sister Wilkins, he said that he found her all upset and that she had fainted before the prison door. He had taken her to his wife's room, and, when she had awakened from the swoon, he had had her sent to the home of Reverend Father Graham, an English minister who had attended *Madame* before she went to the prison. We went to this good man's home in one of the suburbs of Brussels, but he was at that moment in St. Gilles engaged in administering to the last spiritual wants of Miss Cavell. He had obtained this great favour from the German chaplain, who was a kind-hearted and charitable man.

We gathered all these facts from Reverend Graham's housekeeper, and it was in his house that we also found our lost Sister Wilkins.

We waited for about half an hour in that strange and dreary place. It was about ten o'clock when the minister returned. He informed us that *Madame*, our dear mother *Directrice*, was prepared for the terrible ordeal of the morrow. We tried as hard as we possibly could to keep from bursting into tears before the noble-hearted father; we asked him what we could do to help *Madame*. He put on his hat and told us to accompany him to the American Consulate, adding that perhaps the United States Consul might be able to do something.

When we reached the American Consulate, we heard that Mr. Brand Whitlock was ill, but that Mr. Hugh Gibson was ready to receive us. We told that young and noble-minded gentleman our sad story, earnestly entreating him to help us. We certainly must have looked forlorn to him, in that large American room, with tears streaming down our cheeks. It must have moved him to pity, for he immediately volunteered to help us. He sent a hasty message to the Spanish minister, de Villalobar, and one also to the Dutch Ambassador, Maurice Van Hollenhover, for them to assist him in his endeavour to free Miss Cavell. The Dutch ambassador refused to enter the undertaking, but the Spanish Minister, de Villalobar, saddened at the fatal news, came with all possible haste to Mr. Gibson's help. These two gentlemen went together to General Von Bissing's headquarters.

In the meantime, we anxiously awaited the result of their mission seated together in one end of the large room of the Consulate under the protection of the American Eagle that hung, with outspread wings, upon the wall. Our hopes began to rise again; but we were soon doomed to disappointment, however, for when Mr. Gibson and the Spanish Ambassador returned we realized that they, too, were unable to gain any better results than we had done. The Reverend Dr. Graham imparted to us the futile results of their visit to Von Bissing. They found Von Bissing very polite, but he excused himself on the pretext that he was only Governor General of Belgium, and that he did not form part of, or exercise any influence over, the War Council. Consequently he had no say in the affairs of Miss Cavell. Von Bissing phoned, however, to several other German officials for them to use their influence in saving *Madame* from execution; but all in vain! The latter functionaries did not dare to interfere with orders emanating from the German Headquarters of the War Council in Berlin.

General Von Bissing then promised to give Mr. Hugh Gibson a letter of introduction to that most horrible of all men, Von Saubersweig, the most cruel soldier that ever existed. He was Governor of the German War Council in Belgium, and, under his iron rule, had condemned, daily, many an unfortunate person to death or to imprisonment for life.

Mr. Hugh Gibson and the Spanish Ambassador went to this monster's house; but he was absent. They had much difficulty in getting him; but they finally discovered him in a vulgar bar-room where he was relaxing his ferocious mind by viewing entertainments of a low and immoral nature. His Excellency took no pains to conceal his displeasure at being disturbed at his favourite amusements, and at having to be bored again with War Council business. He either found no time to listen to the suppliant voices of the noble gentlemen before him,

131

or, most probably, he was labouring too much under the influence of liquor to be softened by their pleadings; for he immediately became angry, and lost all dignified control over himself. With a flushed face, and a rising voice, he actually screamed at them, that Miss Cavell would be led to execution at four o'clock the next day.

I am ignorant of what further occurred then. Mr. Hugh Gibson has written a book about the judgment of Miss Cavell. It does not enter into the sphere of this humble narrative.

When we heard what these men had to say, we felt that there was no further room left for hope; we turned our sad and weary steps homeward through the dark shadows of that dreary night. It seemed as though we were dragging our unwilling feet over newly made graves.

Upon reaching the *clinique* we found Miss Wilkins in a state of nervous breakdown. We could hear her sad and grave voice praying in a dreary tone, and constantly repeating: "Oh, God! Oh! my Lord! Please give my mistress back to me! Please give my mistress back! Take my life away if you will, but give her back to me"; until, finally, her voice died away in a whisper, and she fell into a state of profound unconsciousness. Her blond hair was so changed that she seemed to have been suddenly transformed into an old woman.

I cannot recollect what we did, Paula, Mania, I and the others, for we did nothing but sob and sob, until our hearts seemed as though they would break.

Towards four o'clock on that fatal morning, we put on our hats and cloaks, and again wended our lonely way through the darkness to the prison. We rang the bell; it struck our ears with a dismal sound that made our souls shiver with horror. When Mr. Marin, the superintendent, opened to us, we halted before the entrance, and exclaimed with voices choked with emotion, "Oh, give her to us! God help us!"

The poor, kind-hearted Mr. Marin had tears in his eyes. He tried to console us by saying that *Madame* was very brave. He learned this much from one of the German wardens, who was, it seemed, more truthful than the others. The superintendent told us that if we waited a while we might possibly catch a glimpse of our beloved mistress, when the automobile would come out of the prison to take her to the "*Tir National*," or rifle range, where she was to be executed.

At five o'clock in the morning, on October the 12th, of memorable date, two hideous war-cars issued grimly from the prison entrance. Anxiously and expectantly we gazed at them. "In which one of these

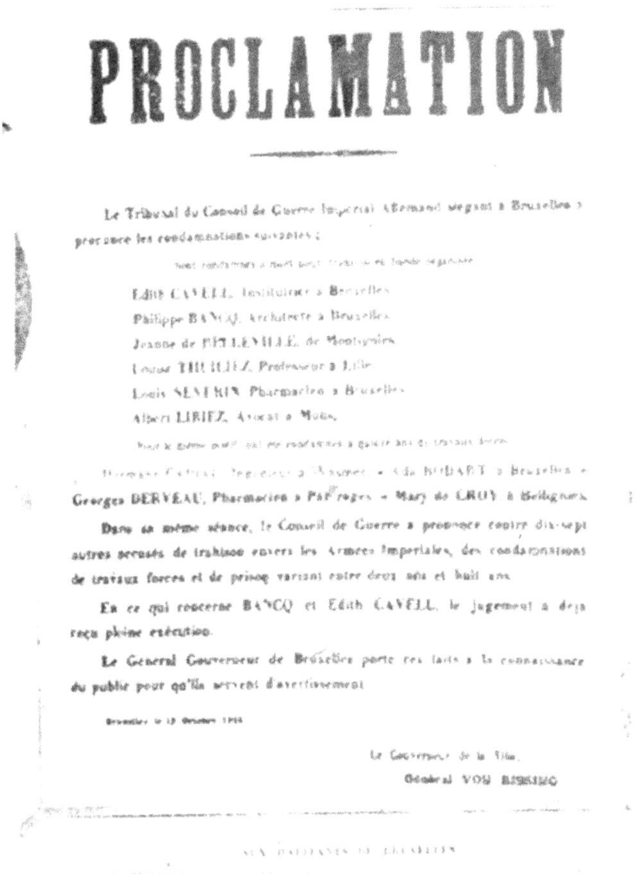

# PROCLAMATION

Le Tribunal du Conseil de Guerre Impérial Allemand siégeant à Bruxelles a prononcé les condamnations suivantes :

[illegible line]

Édith CAVELL, Institutrice à Bruxelles
Philippe BAUCQ, Architecte à Bruxelles
Jeanne de BELLEVILLE, de Montignies
Louise THULIEZ, Professeur à Lille
Louis SÉVERIN, Pharmacien à Bruxelles
Albert LIBIEZ, Avocat à Mons,

[illegible line]

[illegible] — à la HOSTART à Bruxelles —
Georges DERVEAU, Pharmacien à Pâturages — Mary de CROY à Bellignies.

Dans la même séance, le Conseil de Guerre a prononcé contre dix-sept autres accusés de trahison envers les Armées Impériales, des condamnations de travaux forcés et de prison variant entre deux ans et huit ans.

En ce qui concerne BAUCQ et Edith CAVELL, le jugement a déjà reçu pleine exécution.

Le Général Gouverneur de Bruxelles porte ces faits à la connaissance du public pour qu'ils servent d'avertissement.

Bruxelles, le 12 Octobre 1915.

Le Gouverneur de la Ville,
Général VON BISSING

[illegible]

PROCLAMATION ANNOUNCING THE DEATH OF MISS CAVELL

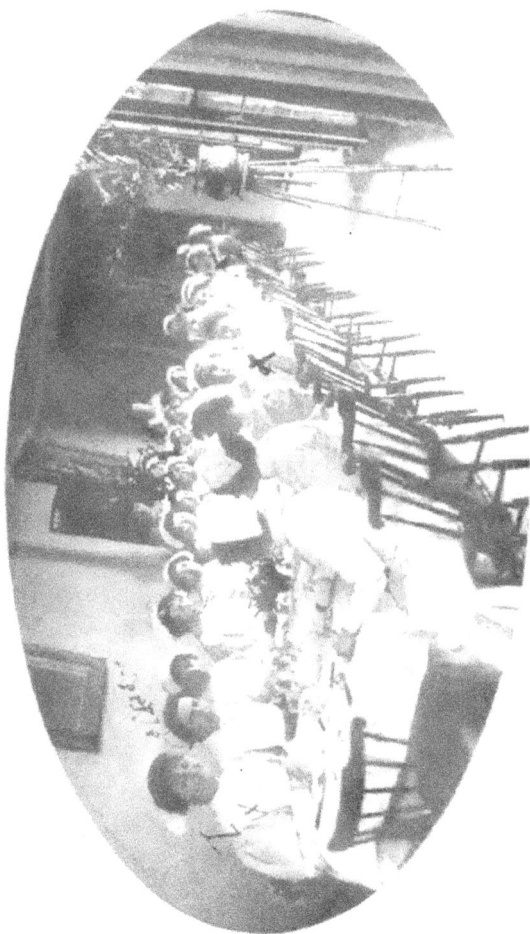

NURSES INDICATED BY CROSS WHO ASSISTED NURSE CAVELL

horrid vehicles was *Madame?*" "In which one was she?"—It seemed to me that I caught sight of her blue uniform. Was it merely imagination, or was it really she?—Who knows?

That was all we saw! The stillness of the city houses seemed to come to our aid. We could only cry out with one voice, "*Madame! Madame!*" as the horrid death-cars rapidly vanished from our tearful eyes.

Without looking any further we mournfully turned our steps towards the New *Clinique*. Upon reaching it, we saw the bright morning sun just pouring its golden beams over a portrait of our *Madame*, surrounded by us nurses. The sight of this picture, crowned as it was with a glorious light, made us keenly feel the sad loss of our martyred Mistress, so suddenly taken away from us. We were racked with sorrow at the thought that we should never see *Madame* again. I could not bear to remain indoors, but went out brooding over her unfortunate fate, thinking only of the cruel German rifles that had ruthlessly murdered her; that the good and kind-hearted woman, whose portrait we just saw, was now lying cold in death, on the forgotten rifle ranges of the "*Tir National!*"

A few hours later on that fatal day of October 12th, we received a final shock, that greatly increased our sorrow and impressed us with the certitude of our irrecoverable loss. Our eyes were assailed by the most pitiless proclamation that we had yet seen, placarded on the walls of Brussels. It read as follows:

Translation of Proclamation;
*Proclamation:*
The Tribunal of the Imperial War Council
of Germany
Held in Brussels
Has pronounced the following sentences;
The following persons are condemned to the penalty of Death for treason in organized bands:
Edith Cavell, a Teacher of Brussels
Philippe Bancq, an Architect of Brussels
Jeanne de Belleville, of Montignies
Louis Thuilliez, a Teacher of Lille
Louis Severin, Pharmacist of Brussels
Albert Libiez, a lawyer of Mons.
For the same motive the following have been condemned to

fifteen years' hard labour;

Herman Capiau, a Civil Engineer of Wasmes

Ada Bodart, of Brussels

George Derveau, a pharmacist of Paturages

Mary de Cröy of Bellignies.

At the same sessions, the War Council has pronounced against seventeen others accused of treason towards the Imperial Armies, sentences of hard-labour, and imprisonment.

As far as concerns Bancq and Edith Cavell, judgment has already been fully executed.

The Governor General of Brussels places these facts before the public as a solemn warning to them.

Governor of the City

General Von Bissing.

Brussels, the 12th Oct., 1915.

### To the Inhabitants of Brussels:

The above is the Proclamation of the Governor Von Bissing, announcing the condemnation to death and the execution of Miss Cavell and of the Architect Bancq, which was placarded on the walls of Brussels in the forenoon of the 12th of October, 1915.

(Exact translation from the facsimile in French.)

From an article entitled *The Last Days of Edith Cavell*.

It is my duty, here, to make some mention of Monsieur Bancq, whose heroic figure merely served as a protest, by having him share the same fate as the great English Martyred Nurse. The only accusation that the Germans could bring against him was that he had printed some articles in *La Libre Belgique*. But I think he had never sheltered a single Englishman in his own home. The brave but unfortunate man left a wife and two children, without any money to help them live during those hard and trying times.

A few days after the execution, Mr. Heeger received from the prison a bundle of clothes which had belonged to our regretted mistress. In it were found her blue jacket, one of the pockets of which contained two sheets of paper. One of them was her last letter to her nurses, and the other consisted of notes and reminiscences of her several trials. In the same package was found the small sum of fifty *francs*. This humble amount was all that she had left, after a life heroically spent in servitude and hardships, in trials and in dangers, a life courageously devoted to the relief of the sick and the care of the dying.

The following is a translation of the last letter of Miss Cavell to her nurses, the original letter being in the possession of The Edith Cavell Clinique, in Brussels.

St. Gilles Prison.

My Dear Nurses:—

This is a very sad moment for me, to write you my last Goodbye. It makes me think of the 17th of September which had closed my eight years as the *Directrice* of our little *clinique*. I was so happy to be called to help in the work our Committee started.

The first of October 1907, we had only four young pupils, now there are many; I believe fifty or sixty counting the trained nurses and the nurses who have left the *clinique*. I have told you very often of the early days; of the difficulties we all had in arranging for your hours of duty, your hours of rest. Everything was new when this work was started in Belgium.

But in a very short time things adjusted themselves. We secured some trained nurses for private cases, some school nurses to work in the public schools of Brussels, the St. Gilles Hospital, the *clinique* of Dr. DePage, the Sanitarium for the treatment of Tuberculosis in Buysinghen, the *clinique* of Dr. Mayer and now many nurses will be called to nurse the wounded soldiers on the battlefields.

When, this last year, our task seemed to diminish, we can find the reason for it in the sad times in which we lived, but, later in our happier days, our work will grow faster in its mighty power.

When I talk to you of the past, it means that it is necessary sometimes to look back to the resolutions we took, and our past experiences should guide us in correcting future errors, that our progress might be greater. In your new *clinique* building you will have many more patients and you will find there I am sure, everything necessary for their comfort as well as for your own also.

It makes me very sad to think that I had not always more time to devote to each of you alone. You all know that I had many occupations, but I hope you will not forget the little talks we had each evening. I told you that voluntary sacrifices would make you happy; that your idea of duty before God and your-self will give you greater support in the sad moments of life and in the face of death.

There are perhaps two or three nurses who remember quite well the little conversations we had together. These nurses should not forget this; having had greater experience, I could see many things clearer and I felt it my duty to show them the right way,

A little word yet—mistrust evil speaking; may I not say this to you?—because I loved my country with my whole heart—I am here. I have seen, in the past eight years and now also, many mistakes which could have been avoided. Here and there, very often, a whispered word, even though uttered without bad in-tention, has many times ruined the good name, the reputation and even the life of somebody.

It is therefore necessary for my nurses to think well before speaking and that you shall cultivate in your life, more loyalty and a holy spirit.

If there is one nurse who has a grievance against me, I beg that she will forgive me. I know that sometimes I have been harsh—too harsh—but never have I been voluntarily unjust and I loved all of you, more than you will ever know.

My fondest wishes for all of you, my young nurses, the nurses who have left the school as well as the nurses who are still there, and I thank you all very much for the kindness, gentleness and courtesy which you have so often shown me.

Truly yours,

Your devoted *Directrice*,

Edith Cavell.

10th October, 1915.

After *Madame* had departed forever from our midst, only a few nurses that had been with her in the old place now remained in the New *Clinique*. We would gather together each evening with our minds constantly drawn towards the Northern section of the town, where the fatal "*Tir National*," with its mournful surroundings, was located. We could see, in imagination, that lonely grave behind the target-numbers of the rifle-range where in winter the icy northern wind would blow, and the scorching sun beat mercilessly down in summer. . . .

In these never-to-be-forgotten times of rugged war and privation we five girls remained steadfastly at the New *Clinique*, of which our dear *Madame* had laid the first stone and for the completion of which she had so ardently worked. . . .

# After-Word

In November, 1918, some days after the Armistice had been signed, the senior nurses of Edith Cavell were called together in one of the parlours of the new building, where three French officers were occupied writing. Without any warning, they thrust two portraits before our startled eyes. They were the photographs of Gaston Quin, and the German who three years before had been hidden in the old *clinique*, and known to us as Mr. X, an Englishman.

We knew Quin at a glance, although his hair had been shorn and he was dressed in prison garb.

These government officials had come to us for information regarding Quin's doings while with us.

We were so utterly confounded at what we saw, and we spoke so mildly among ourselves about him, that the detectives were greatly puzzled at our attitude towards Quin. We burst into tears at the thought that this man who had appeared so innocently to help us, was the real author of all our misfortune. He it was who had helped to betray *Madame*, and had brought trouble and sadness into our young, happy lives!

I cannot well describe what followed this sad and sudden interview with the French law-officers. The story of Quin has been in the newspapers all over the world. As to Quin's ignoble friend, the German whom we called Mr. X, he is far away, probably dead—or murdered perhaps!

In December, 1918, a small group of nurses conducted by some French officers went for the first time to view the humble grave of Miss Cavell. We saw the place of her execution; the wooden fence where Monsieur Bancq awaited his turn to die.

We were struck by the forlorn aspect of the sinister spot, the bleakness and loneliness of the surrounding landscape. There, immediately before our eyes, in all its grim horror, stood the fatal stone where *Madame's* frail form had been supported upon a chair! On that chalky earth, and mud, and rubble which marked her grave, we reverently knelt together as on hallowed ground. . . .

In March, 1919, England claimed the body of the martyred Nurse. *Madame's* sister and her brother-in-law came to the *clinique* to visit the place she had founded, which now bears her name. The King and Queen of the Belgians were present, together with many other notable persons. A solemn ceremony took place, during which a splendid oil-painting of Miss Cavell was placed upon the classroom wall. It was an exact likeness of her as she appeared during the early years of our little school in the *rue de la Culture*. We nurses felt sad at the sight of it. Our heavy hearts carried in them the fond remembrance of this humble woman as she was, when she bravely risked her life and her health, mercifully conducting unfortunate soldiers to safety. . . .

Those times are gone forever; our heroic *Directrice's* young nurses are now scattered far and wide, some are dead, others are trying to forget those terrible days of hardships and of dread. . . .

Little remains for me to add to this narrative. Pauline is a nurse in an English family in Belgium. José has disappeared. Gilles, our faithful guide, went through it all unscathed. He had joined the army after he left us. It was a pleasure to see his honest face, with its laughing blue eyes, radiant with joy at never having been caught by the Boches! Jack, the dog, was some time in José's house, but later, after José's departure, in the house of the Princess De Cröy in France.

In 1920, while I was in Chicago, I read in the papers of the miserable death of Von Saubersweig. Had his mind been tormented by remorse at the thought of the noble victim, whom he had so brutally helped to put to death?

Jacqueline Van Til.

White Plains, N.Y., April 20th, 1921.

141

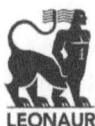